Quintessential Occupational Therapy

A Guide to Areas of Practice

Quintessential Occupational Therapy

A Guide to Areas of Practice

Editor

Robin Akselrud, OTD, OTR/L

Program Director and Professor
Department of Occupational Therapy
Long Island University Brooklyn
Owner
Forward Occupational Therapy PLLC
Brooklyn, New York

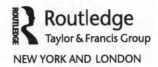

Routledge
Taylor & Francis Group

NEW YORK AND LONDON

First published 2023 by SLACK Incorporated

Published 2024 by Routledge
605 Third Avenue, New York, NY 10158

and by Routledge
4 Park Square, Milton Park, Abingdon, Oxon, OX14 4RN

Routledge is an imprint of the Taylor & Francis Group, an informa business

Library of Congress Control Number: 2022060963

Cover: Lori Shields

ISBN: 9781630918194 (pbk)
ISBN: 9781003526230 (ebk)

DOI: 10.4324/9781003526230

Dedication

This book is dedicated to my current, past, and future students. This book was written in your honor. Your dedication, motivation, sleepless nights, tears, and fears were all worth it. We are part of a profession that has NO boundaries. Occupational therapists can do anything and everything. There is so much opportunity for you for growth and innovation within our profession. I hope this book excites you and helps you envision your bright future. You got this!

Contents

Section I: Established Practice Areas

Section II: Emerging Practice Areas

Acknowledgments

This book would not be in your hands right now without the support and assistance of so many.

I would like to thank my husband, Yossi, and my children, Moshe, Reeva, and Elie. Your love and support for my ideas is what drives me to create even more. I love you!

To my parents, for always believing in me, even when others doubted my abilities.

To my in-laws, for their support and cheerleading throughout this process.

To Jacqueline Monroe, for all that you do for my children.

To the contributing authors in this book, many of whom I have never met in person. Thank you so much for your time, knowledge, and excitement over this project!

To my colleagues at Long Island University Brooklyn and Hofstra University, who listen and smile at all my ideas and then give great feedback.

To my professors at Quinnipiac University, for inspiring my mediocre self to become an agent of change within the occupational therapy profession.

To Brien Cummings, who "walked" me through this process from beginning to end.

To my students, for providing me with daily inspiration and for taking this "ride" with me as a first-time author. I hope that this book is exactly what you have been waiting for!

About the Editor

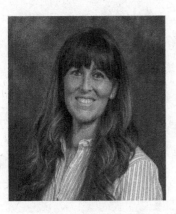

Robin Akselrud, OTD, OTR/L, received her Bachelor of Science/Master of Science degree from Touro College and her Post-Professional Doctorate from Quinnipiac University in 2017. She is the program director and an assistant professor at Long Island University–Brooklyn in the Bachelor of Science/Master of Science Occupational Therapy program. Dr. Akselrud was an assistant professor and academic fieldwork coordinator at Hofstra University from 2017 to 2020 and was an adjunct professor at Long Island University–Brooklyn, Touro College, and York College from 2012 to 2018.

Dr. Akselrud is a Certified Early Intervention provider. In 2010, she established an outpatient occupational therapy private practice, Forward Occupational Therapy PLLC.

In 2021, she published a self-development planner for students and practitioners, *The My OT Journey Planner.* Dr. Akselrud has also developed the "My OT Journey" podcast, a student-run podcast platform to facilitate unity, communication, and leadership skills amongst occupational therapy students.

Dr. Akselrud is currently in her second term as the leadership and management coordinator for the American Occupational Therapy Association Home and Community Health Special Interest Section and a member of the Association of Schools Advancing Health Professions Leadership Committee. Dr. Akselrud's research is focused on interprofessional collaboration and working with mothers to support their own physical and mental health and their children's development.

Contributing Authors

Inna Babaeva, PhD, OTR/L (Chapter 9)
Occupational Therapist
Lighthouse Guild
New York, New York

James Battaglia, EdD, OTR/L, CHT (Chapter 3)
Rehabilitation Supervisor
Northwell Health Sports Therapy and
Rehabilitation Services
East Meadow, New York

Aviva Blaustein, MS, OTR/L, CAPS (Chapter 1)
Clinical Specialist
Occupational Therapy
Rusk Rehabilitation
New York University Langone Health
New York, New York

Gioia J. Ciani, MS, OTD, OTR/L (Chapter 11)
Faculty
Occupational Therapy Program
Hofstra University
Long Island, New York

Dale A. Coffin, EdD, OTR/L (Chapter 5)
Stony Brook University
Stony Brook, New York

Shelli Dry, OTD, OTR/L, MEd (Chapter 16)
Vice President of Clinical Care
HelloHero
Southampton, New York

Nicole A. Fidanza, OTD, OTR/L (Chapter 4)
Clinical Assistant Professor
Quinnipiac University
Hamden, Connecticut

Melanie C. Frank-Hirsch, OTR (Chapter 4)
Director of Rehabilitation
A. Holly Patterson Extended Care Facility
Nassau Health Care Corporation
East Meadow, New York

Dana Fried, MOT, OTR/L (Chapter 1)
Occupational Therapist
Long Island, New York

Mindy Garfinkel, OTD, OTR/L, ATP
(Chapter 14)
Assistant Program Director and Associate
Professor
Occupational Therapy Doctorate Program
Yeshiva University
New York, New York

Melissa K. Gerber, OTD, OTR/L (Chapter 6)
Great Neck Public Schools
Speaker
Therapeutic Service Incorporated
Education Resources Incorporated
Owner/President
4MYKIDSOTPC
Great Neck, New York

Heather Gilbert, MS, OTR/L (Chapter 8)
Post-Professional Doctor of Occupational
Therapy Candidate
Part-Time Lecturer
Tufts University
Medford, Massachusetts
Adjunct Faculty
University of New Hampshire
Durham, New Hampshire

Clarice Grote, MS, OTR/L (Chapter 7)
CEO and Medicare Specialist
Amplify OT
Durham, North Carolina

Nicola Grun, MOTR/L (Chapter 7)
Occupational Therapist
Two Trees Physical Therapy
Oxnard, California

Kristy Gulotta, MS, OTR/L, BCMH, CGCP
(Chapter 8)
Behavioral Health Occupational Therapist
Northwell Health
Cochair
1 North/1 East Collaborative Care Council
Mental Health Lecturer
Great Neck, New York

Henry Hanif, MA, OTR/L (Chapter 8)
Senior Occupational Therapist
Mount Sinai Beth Israel Hospital
Adjunct Faculty
Long Island University
New York University
Touro College
SUNY Downstate
New York

Brett Herman, MS, OTR/L, BCG, LSVT
(Chapter 7)
QAPD Clinical Specialist
FOX Rehabilitation
Philadelphia, Pennsylvania

Yu-Pin Hsu, EdD, OTR/L (Chapter 9)
Hofstra University
Lighthouse Guild
New York

Douglene Jackson, PhD, OTR/L, LMT, ATP,
CYT, FAOTA (Chapter 10)
Founder
GIFTS Institute

LoriBeth Kimmel, MS, OTR (Chapter 5)
Pediatric Occupational Therapy
Early Intervention
New Jersey

Ivelisse Lazzarini, EdD, OTD, OTR/L
(Chapter 11)
Interim Program Director
College of Graduate & Professional Studies
Occupational Therapy Department
Notre Dame of Maryland University
Baltimore, Maryland

Catherine J. Leslie, PhD, OTR/L, MOT, CEIS
(Chapter 5)
MGH Institute of Health Professions
Charlestown, Massachusetts

Rachelle Lydell, MSOT, OTR/L
(Chapters 5 and 10)
Occupational Therapist
Owner and Founder
Vive Therapeutic Services LLC
Park Ridge, Illinois

Jacqueline Ndwaru McGlamery, OTD, OT/L,
CCM, ECHM (Chapter 7)
Owner and Founder
First Coast Aging in Place Solutions
Jacksonville, Florida

April O'Connell, OT/L, CHT, ACSM (Chapter 3)
Clinical Specialist
New York University Langone Health
New York, New York

AnneMarie O'Hearn, MEd, MPA (Chapter 9)
Vice President Education and Training
Lighthouse Guild
New York, New York

Heather Page, OTD, OTR/L (Chapter 5)
Pediatric Occupational Therapist
Thom Springfield Infant Toddler Services
Springfield, Massachusetts

Michelle M. Rampulla, MS, OTR/L, CPRP
(Chapter 8)
Occupational Therapist
Penn Foundation, Inc.
St. Luke's University Health Network
Easton, Pennsylvania

Miriam Ringel, OTR/L (Chapter 1)
Rusk Rehabilitation
New York University Langone Health
New York, New York

Taylor Skoller, MS, OTR/L (Chapter 1)
Occupational Therapist
Long Island, New York

Esty Spitzer, OTD, OTR/L (Chapter 2)
Turning Point OT
Brooklyn, New York
Adjunct Professor
Occupational Therapy Department
Yeshiva University
New York, New York

*Teresa (Tee) Stock, OTD, MSOT, MBA, OTR/L
(Chapters 6, 12, and 17)*
Occupational Therapist
Tee Stock Pediatric OT
Needham, Massachusetts

Kelsey Swope, MOT, OTR/L, BCG (Chapter 7)
Alvernia University
Reading, Pennsylvania

*Miriam Wachspress, MS, OTR/L
(Chapters 12 and 15)*
Amistad Dual Language School
New York City Department of Education
New York, New York

Lee Westover, MS, OTR/L (Chapter 13)
Occupational Therapist
Clinical Fieldwork Instructor
New York, New York

Anna Wold, OTR/L (Chapter 15)
Occupational Therapist
Craniosacral Therapist
Monsey, New York

Introduction

I truly love the occupational therapy profession. And what I love the most about my profession of choice are the many different areas of practice.

My Career Path

When I started my career journey more than 15 years ago, I chose to work in school-based practice, and then after a year in the field, I chose to work in early intervention in the after school hours. I enjoyed working in pediatric practice, but after another a few months, I decided to add some geriatric home health visits to my schedule. The balance of school-based, pediatric, and geriatric practice felt like a great balance, that is until 7 years later when I decided that I wanted to open a private practice—and I did! After establishing my private practice, I became a consultant for a primary care facility and added occupational therapy to their variety of treating providers.

Sadly, when rates for insurance reimbursement plummeted and quality of care was compromised, I decided that academic education was my next step. As an assistant professor, I gained a new view of my career trajectory and a deeper understanding of my passions. Today I am a full-time professor, author, and podcaster ("My OT Journey"), and I still carve out some treatment time for my infants and toddlers in early intervention. I am sharing my career journey with the hope that you, the readers, will also explore your true passions in your occupational therapy practice, and that is exactly why I created this book.

How to Use This Book

Have you ever wondered what it would be like to work in a different area of practice? Have you ever thought about switching practice areas but were too nervous or fearful to make the "jump"? This book contains 17 chapters that focus on what to expect in a variety of practice settings. Each chapter is written by specialists in the field who want to share their knowledge and experiences with you. In this text, you will discover typical daily schedules and caseload expectations in various settings, samples of documentation, case studies, and helpful resources and tips for entering each practice area.

#OTRocks—and I hope that you enjoy this book and your own occupational therapy career journey!

Section I

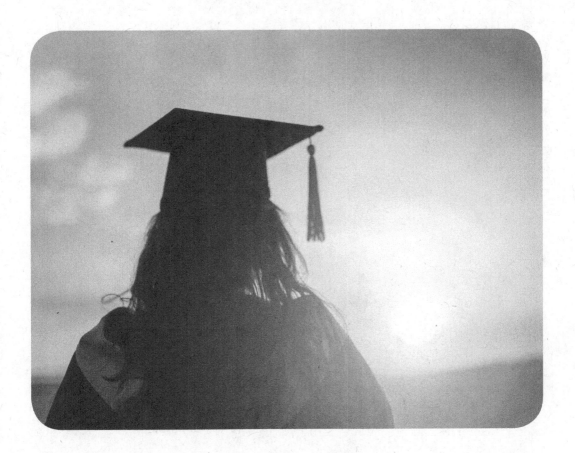

ESTABLISHED PRACTICE AREAS

1

Hospital-Based Rehabilitation

*Miriam Ringel, OTR/L; Aviva Blaustein, MS, OTR/L, CAPS;
Dana Fried, MOT, OTR/L; and Taylor Skoller, MS, OTR/L*

ACUTE CARE

Miriam Ringel, OTR/L and Aviva Blaustein, MS, OTR/L, CAPS

Acute Care in a Nutshell

Acute care is an inpatient hospital setting for patients with critical medical conditions. These patients are admitted to the hospital for management of a sudden decline in medical or functional status resulting from a traumatic event, exacerbation of a progressive or existing disease, or the development of a new condition.

The medical team's goal during acute care is to manage life-threatening and critical issues. For patients who are medically stable, the team's focus shifts to promoting functional independence. Occupational therapists have a unique role on the acute care team, providing interventions to improve functional status and prevent physical and cognitive complications resulting from immobility or disease-related decline. Occupational therapy is the only health care spending category that has been shown to reduce hospital readmissions (Rogers et al., 2016) through facilitating early mobilization, restoring function, preventing further decline, and coordinating care, including transition and discharge planning (American Occupational Therapy Association [AOTA], 2017).

Akselrud, R. (Ed.). *Quintessential Occupational Therapy:
A Guide to Areas of Practice* (pp 3-14).
© 2023 Taylor & Francis Group.

Evaluation and Assessments

An occupational therapy evaluation in acute care is untimed but typically ranges from 30 to 45 minutes. Therefore, assessments seek to gain a broad perspective and less detailed-oriented description of a patient's abilities and limitations. For example, goniometry is not used to measure specific degrees of motion; rather, motion is assessed only as it relates to function (e.g., 1/2 range right shoulder flexion and its impact on upper body dressing).

Some common standardized assessments and tools used by occupational therapists in acute care are as follows:

- The Boston University Activity Measure for Post Acute Care short form for basic mobility, daily activity, and applied cognition (Jette et al., 2017)
- The Confusion Assessment Method for the Intensive Care Unit (Inouye, 1998)
- The Functional Independence Measure (Keith et al., 1987) or Quality Indicator (American Speech-Language-Hearing Association, 2006) scales

Interventions

In the acute care setting, occupational therapists' responsibilities include promoting early mobilization and positioning for skin protection to prevent breakdown and pressure injury, as well as evaluating the need for splints and fabricating orthoses to preserve joint integrity. Therapists perform bedside training for safety and independence with transfers and mobility, especially for patients with changes in weight-bearing status. Interventions also include training in self-care activities (e.g., bathing, dressing) with adaptive devices as needed and teaching safe eating and swallowing techniques. Therapists use neuromuscular reeducation, trunk stabilization, and balance activities to improve patients' bed mobility, activities of daily living (ADLs) and instrumental activities of daily living (IADLs), and postural control. For patients who are more dependent, sessions focus on caregiver training with friends, family members, or partners to assist with home exercise programs (HEP), range of motion (ROM) exercises, and skin checks, as well as diagnosis-specific education. The overall goal of occupational therapy in acute care is to assess a patient's level of independence and impairments to facilitate a safe discharge plan to the next level of care.

Discharge Planning

The interdisciplinary team discusses the discharge disposition for patients who are medically stable and ready for the next care level. The decision is based on multiple factors, including diagnosis, prognosis, home set-up, available social support, current functional status, and insurance authorization and coverage. For patients who require additional rehabilitation, training, and education, discharge options include acute rehabilitation, sometimes referred to as inpatient rehabilitation, in a hospital or subacute rehabilitation in a skilled nursing facility. The differences between these two levels are described in later sections.

Patients who can be mobilized safely either via the assistance of available caregivers or who are ambulatory and do not require daily skilled nursing care can be discharged to home. Often, these patients are discharged with either follow-up home care services or outpatient rehabilitation visits.

It was determined that Jack was unable to return home at this point, as he lives alone and is not at his prior level of function. He requires moderate assistance to perform his basic ADLs due to impaired balance and right-side hemiparesis, and safety concerns remain, as Jack requires assistance of another person with basic mobility to the bathroom. Jack was motivated to participate and worked hard in his bedside therapies in the hospital. Therefore, he is a candidate for acute rehabilitation, and after obtaining insurance authorization, Jack was accepted in the inpatient rehabilitation unit in the hospital.

Tips and Advice From the Field

Caseload and Schedule

Hospital schedules can vary; however, a typical day for an acute care occupational therapist is about 8 hours, usually beginning in the morning around 7:30 a.m. to 8:30 a.m. and ending around 3:30 p.m. to 4:30 p.m. Some hospitals have flexed shifts (e.g., Tuesday through Saturday, Sunday through Thursday) to cover weekend days, and some have shifts ending around 7:00 p.m. to cover patients undergoing surgery later in the day. A caseload productivity expectation is generally 7 to 10 patients per day and can depend on the number of assigned initial patient evaluations or medical complexity.

Mentorship

For new graduates, especially those without acute care fieldwork experience, guidance and mentorship are required. These are especially important due to the risks of working with medically complex and dependent patients with myriad safety and mobility precautions. Because of the structure of the acute care setting, another occupational therapy clinician may not be available in the nearby vicinity or at all times for assistance or questions. The work is fast paced, and the schedule is fluid depending on the patient's medical status and when they are available to be seen.

Acute Inpatient Rehabilitation in a Nutshell

An *inpatient rehabilitation facility* or *acute rehabilitation* is a rigorous therapy program in a hospital setting characterized by the provision of 15 hours of therapy per 7 consecutive days or 1 week, generally consisting of 3 hours per day for at least 5 days per week. Patients are expected to reasonably tolerate this intensive therapy schedule and can actively participate and significantly benefit from this program, making measurable and functional gains within a realistic timeframe. The standard of therapy care is generally one-on-one therapy, and to qualify for acute rehabilitation, a patient must require the ongoing intervention of multiple therapy disciplines (e.g., physical therapy, occupational therapy, or speech-language pathology; Centers for Medicare & Medicaid Services [CMS], 2018).

Typically, patients in this setting have a neurological diagnosis of cerebrovascular accident, tumor, trauma, epilepsy, spinal cord injury, Parkinson's disease, or multiple sclerosis. Other diagnoses include general deconditioning, disorders of consciousness, oncological or cardiac diseases, or orthopedic issues and amputations.

Acute rehabilitation requires physician supervision and the collaborative coordination of an interdisciplinary team. Team conferences are held once a week for each patient, beginning at the date of admission. This team must include a physician, nurse, social worker or case manager, and a licensed therapist from each discipline involved in a patient's treatment. The team meets to discuss patient medical updates, progress toward goals, barriers to discharge, resolutions to problems impeding progress, monitoring and revising the treatment plan and team goals as necessary, and discharge planning (CMS, 2012).

Evaluation and Assessments

Jack is admitted to acute rehabilitation on May 21st. On May 22nd, the occupational therapist performs Jack's initial evaluation. She assesses his vital signs before and after the evaluation, as well as his alertness and orientation, bed mobility, static and dynamic sitting–standing balance, cognition, vision, ROM, manual muscle testing (MMT) score, sensation, tone, reflexes, coordination, serial opposition, proprioception, kinesthesia, perceptual skills (e.g., neglect, apraxia, ability to judge distance), and ADLs and IADLs performance.

Some common assessments used in acute rehabilitation include the Functional Independence Measure or Quality Indicator scales according to CMS guidelines, as well as various domain-specific measures, such as the following:

- *Cognition*: Montreal Cognitive Assessment (Nasreddine et al., 2005), Toglia Contextual Memory Test (Toglia, 1993), Loewenstein Occupational Therapy Cognitive Assessment (Katz et al., 2002), and Moss Attention Rating Scale (Whyte et al., 2003)
- *Vision*: General screens, confrontation visual field testing, and stereopsis tests
- *Perception*: Kessler Foundation Neglect Assessment Process, Behavioral Inattention Test (Menon & Korner-Bitensky, 2004), Bells Test (Gauthier et al., 1989), and Test of Upper Limb Apraxia (Vanbellingen et al., 2010)
- *Motor*: ROM, MMT, Modified Ashworth Scale (MAS; Harb & Kishner, 2022), dynamometer, pinch meter, and 9-Hole Peg Test (Mathiowetz et al., 1985b)
- *Sensation*: Light touch, two-point discrimination, sharp/dull discrimination, and the American Spinal Cord Injury Association Impairment Scale (Roberts et al., 2017)

Interventions

Treatment in this setting is focused on discharging the patient safely and preferably returning to home. Sessions focus on retraining patients to perform ADLs and IADLs as independently as possible targeting any deficit areas highlighted in the initial evaluations. This approach is both rehabilitative to specific areas of limitation and compensatory depending on whether the possibility of recovery exists or if the full recovery will take longer than the rehabilitation length of stay will permit.

The interdisciplinary team is particularly important when designing treatment sessions and approaches for patients. The team's physicians may tweak medication and seek feedback on patient behavior, including agitation and restlessness or arousal in sessions, episodes of seizure, or any changes occurring in muscle tone. Neuropsychologists may develop a behavioral plan for patients who are challenging or inappropriate. Neuro-optometrists may recommend vision strategies and prescribe prisms for eye malalignments postinjury. Speech therapists may recommend cognitive protocols or a special diet to use during feeding tasks, and physical therapists may provide input on optimal mobility techniques. Occupational therapists can use these recommendations and relay information about additional suggestions for or feedback on patient performance during their session.

Interventions include working on self-care activities (e.g., grooming, bathing, dressing) with use of adaptive equipment (AE) or durable medical equipment and assistive technology and devices as needed. Patients may need AE or durable medical equipment after discharge, and occupational therapists can order the equipment, as well as write a letter of medical necessity, to ensure insurance coverage for equipment, such as hospital beds and wheelchair seating and management. Therapists also focus on mobility, safe transfers, and training for postsurgical protocols, including for appropriate weight-bearing and precautions.

Occupational therapy sessions can include neuromuscular reeducation via manual techniques, electrical stimulation, kinesio tape, and robotic-assisted devices, as well as evaluating the need for and fabricating splints to maintain joint integrity and prevent skin breakdown in the event of muscle tone changes. Therapists can also introduce assistive technology such as call bells, mobile devices, or tablets to communicate and use for other desirable activities. Vision exercises can be implemented, including trialing the use of prisms if prescribed by the neuro-optometrist. The treatment plan may include working on community mobility, home management, and meal preparation, if applicable. Throughout the stay, therapists can target cognitive and perceptual deficits, including training for using compensatory techniques on discharge.

Discharge Planning

The ultimate goal of acute rehabilitation is for patients to return to home and the community. The rehabilitation team holds family meetings when necessary to discuss a patient's current status, progress thus far, and plans for discharge. This is a time when the team determines a need for skilled caregiver training by all disciplines on effective and safe patient care, including performing prescribed HEP prior to a patient leaving the hospital. Thus, occupational therapists are a significant part of the safe discharge planning process.

For patients who are able to return home with appropriate support and equipment, the discharge to home is usually accompanied by follow-up home visits or patient visits to an outpatient facility. A typical length of stay during acute rehabilitation is about 2 to 3 weeks depending on diagnosis. For patients unable to return to their prior living setting within that timeframe or if no safe discharge is available in the community, patients will transition to the next level of care in a subacute rehabilitation facility.

Subacute Rehabilitation in a Nutshell

Subacute care, which is less intensive than acute rehabilitation, usually provides a combination of physical, occupational, and speech therapies; however, the number of therapy hours is lower than that during acute rehabilitation, ranging from 1 to 2 hours per day. The average length of stay at a subacute facility is generally longer than at an inpatient rehabilitation facility. While the therapy is less intense, patients are usually afforded more time to participate in the rehabilitation process.

Occupational therapy services in a subacute setting might include task simplification for ADLs, energy conservation to prevent fatigue, education on how to use AE, weight-bearing precautions, and many of the same interventions used in acute rehabilitation, providing the facility has the same equipment and resources. Interventions are designed to facilitate each patient to return safely back to former occupational roles.

Tips and Advice From the Field

Caseload

In the acute rehabilitation setting, an occupational therapist practitioner will typically see five to six patients per day for 1 to 1.5 hours. There is a strong team approach to care, and occupational therapists closely collaborate with other team members, including speech-language pathologists, physical therapists, nurses, physicians, social workers, and patients' families or caregivers.

Suitability for Practice

Acute and subacute rehabilitation are both ideal settings for new occupational therapy graduates looking to expand their skill set, knowledge base, and clinical competency. While the work can be demanding and challenging, serving on the interdisciplinary team in a hospital setting can be fulfilling, stimulating, and exhilarating.

Continuing Education and Resources

Continuing education is imperative to stay current with evidence and best practice. There are many options for expanding your knowledge base and expertise. Depending on your interests, you can obtain certifications in specialty areas (i.e., kinesio taping, assistive technology, stroke or brain injury specialization). The AOTA is a great resource to find these courses and access research, events, courses, and other materials.

OUTPATIENT REHABILITATION

Dana Fried, MOT, OTR/L and Taylor Skoller, MS, OTR/L

Outpatient Rehabilitation in a Nutshell

Clients who require additional skilled occupational therapy services following inpatient, sub-acute, or home care services may be recommended for *outpatient rehabilitation services*. Individuals may also receive outpatient services if the severity of the injury does not require hospitalization. In an outpatient facility, clients are typically seen one to three times per week, although the number may vary based on patient symptomatology.

Patients in outpatient facilities will present for treatment with an array of diagnoses. The population referred to and seen for services in a facility depends on the niche in which the facility specializes as well as the specialties and certifications of the employed therapists.

In neurorehabilitation, typical diagnoses seen include cerebrovascular accident, such as anoxic, hypoxic, or traumatic brain injuries; encephalopathy; brain tumors; Parkinson's disease; or multiple sclerosis. Skills addressed in treatment include strategies for any physical, cognitive, visual, perceptual, or emotional deficits affecting occupational participation.

For physical capacity deficits, a patient experiencing a neurological event may require interventions to address ROM, muscle strength, motor-praxis, and coordination skills. In addition, patients may require interventions for reduced visual skills, including but not limited to oculomotor skills and visual field changes, scanning, and perception. Basic cognitive to complex executive functioning skills may be affected depending on brain injury. Skills addressed in treatment can range from basic orientation, sustained attention, working memory, and sequencing skills to more complex metacognition, divided attention, reasoning skills, and planning and prioritization.

The setting is dependent on not only the facility's specialty but also on the occupational therapist's area of expertise. For occupational therapists who are certified hand therapists (CHTs) or certified lymphedema therapists, the setting's clientele would reflect their area of practice. For example, CHTs may address various orthopedic injuries in the upper extremity.

Evaluation and Assessments

Before conducting an initial evaluation, occupational therapists review all received medical records, including reports from inpatient hospitalization, evaluation and treatment notes from various disciplines, and imaging results. If any pertinent information is not available (e.g., clearance for specified physical activity), then the therapist contacts the referring physician directly to learn about a patient's current physical abilities and limitations.

At the start of an evaluation, occupational therapists conduct a client interview to learn past medical history or that of the current illness or event, including any previous courses of rehabilitation, prior level of function, current functional status, and client and caregiver treatment goals. A vital clinical skill is to incorporate follow-up questions throughout the evaluation process to gain an accurate picture of a patient's functionality. Further patient complaints may present themselves as their performance skills are challenged. Inconsistencies with objective measures and self-report can lead to further development of how a patient is truly functioning.

After the patient interview, occupational therapists perform objective measurements and select setting-dependent screening and evaluation tools. Therapists record both passive ROM (PROM) and active ROM (AROM) at applicable joint planes via goniometry. ROM is an essential prerequisite to determine appropriateness of further muscle testing and assign a proper grading recording during the evaluation process.

Once AROM and PROM are determined, occupational therapists assess muscle strength utilizing MMT. Muscle strength testing can be quantified by a numerical grade (0 to 5) or a qualifying descriptor that provides a measurement of the degree of weakness at the corresponding muscle or muscle groups (Flinn et al., 2008). The Break Test is a commonly used technique involving having the patient hold an isometric muscle contraction at the point of a muscle's greatest mechanical advantage (Flinn et al., 2008). Providing proper stabilization and resistive force are essential for determining where the isometric contraction is unable to hold against the resistance provided. Muscle strength testing can also be determined via ROM in a gravity-eliminated position or against gravity, which is an isotonic contraction without resistance (Flinn et al., 2008).

Dynamometer testing is another measure for muscle strength, specifically at the hand. Grip strength is recorded after a 1- to 2-second timeframe to build up muscle strength and provide a hold to maximize strength implementation over multiple trials (Flinn et al., 2008). Patients provide three maximum voluntary contractions that are averaged and compared to normative standards (Beebe & Lang, 2009). Spasticity, which is velocity dependent, is measured via the MAS, which ranges from 0 (no increase in muscle tone) to 4 (affected part[s] rigid; Bohannon & Smith, 1987).

A variety of assessments are available for upper extremity motor function. One test commonly used for manual dexterity and gross motor coordination is the Box and Block Test, which has a goal of transferring as many blocks as possible over a midline partition in a 1-minute time period (Mathiowetz et al., 1985a). Fine motor coordination measures may include but are not limited to the 9-Hole Peg Test, Purdue Pegboard Test, and Grooved Pegboard. These tests can provide quantitative data to determine a patient's current skill level and help determine the effectiveness of skilled treatment services provided (Lang et al., 2013). Recording patient scores at baseline and again at reevaluation helps provide evidence as to why skilled occupational therapy services are recommended or should be discontinued.

Standardized assessments are used throughout outpatient practice to meet a patient's varying needs and include the following:

- The Fugl-Meyer Assessment to evaluate physical needs (Gladstone et al, 2002)
- The Dynamic Loewenstein Occupational Therapy Cognitive Assessment to evaluate visual and cognitive needs (Katz et al., 2002)
- The Behavioural Assessment of Dysexecutive Syndrome to evaluate higher level executive functioning skills (Wilson et al., 1996)

The timing of progress evaluations can depend on a patient's health insurance coverage, as well as clinical recommendations for both short- and long-term goals. These reports allow occupational therapists to reevaluate ADLs performance skills and functional status to justify the need for continued skilled services or whether discharge is appropriate. A discharge summary is completed at the termination of services and includes new measurements related to established goals, as well as any recommendations for post discharge participation, which may include continued engagement in HEPs, transition to community programming or a support group, or participation in vocational training or volunteer exploration.

Jill is a 23-year-old female who was in college and working part-time in construction. Jill experienced a traumatic brain injury following a fall at work. She received extensive medical treatment, and when deemed medically stable and safe for discharge from inpatient care to home with family, Jill was referred to outpatient occupational therapy for an evaluation. Jill's chief complaint included reduced functional use of her left hand and a goal of returning to school and work in the future. Upon evaluation, occupational independence was discussed with Jill and her family to gain insight into areas of difficulty and subjective reports of performance. Physical measures were completed, as described in this section, which indicated reduced dominant, left upper extremity AROM, grip strength, motor-praxis skills, and coordination. In regards to cognitive skills, a standardized scheduling task at school-age level was completed indicating reduced organization, attention to detail, and logical reasoning. Jill also presented with left-sided visual deficits, impacting both her safety and independence at home, in the community, and for successful work/school reintegration at that time. Areas of difficulty were discussed at evaluation and goals were established with Jill and her family based on reported complaints and demonstrated deficits impacting safety and functional independence in ADLs.

Interventions

Depending on their clinical caseload, facility's clientele, and policies, occupational therapists may see 6 to 12 patients on a given day. In addition to evaluating and treating patients, occupational therapists may have other job duties and responsibilities, including phone interactions such as contacting physicians to obtain relevant medical information and reaching out to clients and caregivers to carry over recommendations (e.g., purchasing AE). Meetings with clients, families, and case managers occur as needed to update respective parties on patient progress or barriers to rehabilitation, as well as to establish an appropriate discharge plan. The workload includes peer chart reviews to ensure that medical records are correct and complete. In-service training on community resources and related continuing education courses may be available as well.

Full-time occupational therapy practice in an outpatient setting typically involves working Monday through Friday for 7.5 to 8 hour days. The work schedule can vary because some facilities have early morning hours, and some begin treatment later in the day. As patients may have family and work responsibilities, physician appointments, or other commitments within their daily schedules, flexible outpatient rehabilitation times allow patients to schedule appointments according to their own needs. As such, some facilities may offer weekend hours, with a work week of 5 varied days in this setting (e.g., Tuesday through Saturday), or a 4-day work week with longer days. Offering earlier or later therapy sessions allows patients to participate in therapy before or after work.

Schedules of per diem occupational therapists can vary depending with the outpatient facility's requirements. This type of practitioner may be needed for coverage for absent full-time employees or to manage an additional caseload due to a high patient volume. Hours are flexible and can fluctuate from a couple of hours to a half day to a full day. Because the work is nonstandardized, per diem clinicians may be able to hold more than one per diem job at a time.

Outpatient occupational therapy sessions can range from 30 to 90 minutes. Sessions may be one-on-one for patients with severe deficits who require more direct hands-on attention or may be doubled sessions for patients who benefit from both direct and indirect treatment time. Scheduling also depends on a patient's insurance coverage. Occupational therapy initial evaluations can range from 30 to 60 minutes depending on complexity. Progress reports and discharges are the same length as a standard treatment session.

Group sessions are available for patients who may benefit from peer interaction, group dynamics, or simulation of community experiences. Cognitive skills or impairments can be targeted during group therapy sessions, as well as performance skills. For example, a clinician leading an attention skills group may focus on the hierarchical levels of attention; focusing on these skills in a social and dynamic environment can help facilitate community reintegration and resumption of complex ADLs and IADLs.

Interventions in outpatient settings are a continuation of the services provided in inpatient, subacute, or home services. The overarching goal is to maximize safety and functional independence in all aspects of patients' lives, which may include occupational engagement in the home, at work, or in the community. Occupational therapists may also provide community resources to maximize support.

Treatment sessions involve remediation of deficits, as well as provision of adaptations to improve a patient's independence level. The focus is on generalization and the carry over of skills to functional practice in the patient's context. Adjusting or modifying sessions is key to addressing individual patient needs. Tasks can require upgrades, downgrades, or adaptations to meet the just-right challenge to maximize patient success and target the most pertinent goals.

Jill's course of outpatient treatment focused on improving the functional use of her left upper extremity, visual attention to the left side, and cognitive skills in order to facilitate successful reintegration into the school, work, and community settings. Various treatment activities included computer tasks to simulate return to school and environmental awareness tasks to simulate demands for return to work. Client was also educated on and implemented strategies to incorporate the affected nondominant left upper extremity into ADLs, including stabilization of clothing during fastener management. Jill and her mother were educated on strategies to increase attention to the left side, including use of the Lighthouse Strategy, to ensure increased safety during functional ambulation and to promote maximal independence. Jill was referred to a neuro-optometrist during her course of therapy for vision therapy and a physiatrist for pain management of her left upper extremity.

Discharge Planning

From the time an occupational therapist is meeting a client for an initial evaluation, discharging planning has begun. The goal of any course of treatment is always to facilitate safe reintegration into the home and community. Prior to discharging a client, the client's goals and progress are reviewed with the client and caregiver, if applicable. HEP will be reviewed and/or upgraded, community resources will be dispensed (e.g., psychosocial support groups), and education on any pieces of AE or compensatory strategies will be complete. If applicable, continued skilled occupational therapy services will be recommended elsewhere, whether it is with the shift of focus to maintenance therapy or for future services if the client has a progressive condition.

Progress evaluations were completed at regular intervals to determine improvements toward goals set forth and continued clinical need. Jill demonstrated significant improved performance in functional use of her nondominant left upper extremity to incorporate into all bilateral tasks for basic ADLs performance. Left-sided visual deficits persisted; however, Jill demonstrated ability to implement compensatory strategies with supervision. Overtime, Jill plateaued in improvements toward physical, cognitive, visual, and functional goals set forth. Discharge planning occurred with Jill, Jill's parents (as per her consent), and Jill's case worker. Communication with the interdisciplinary team consistently occurred and based on Jill's functional ambulation difficulties determined by physical therapy and visual deficits in conjunction with reduced processing speed, all parties were in agreement that return to construction work in the previous capacity would not be safe at that time. With the assistance of family and professional support, Jill began participation in an acquired brain inquiry educational program as a prerequisite and to prepare further for school reintegration. Her occupational therapist also connected Jill with a community brain injury support group for recreational and volunteer opportunities. This also offered her connections to other individuals in the community who had experienced similar injuries. Jill's HEP was consistently updated throughout the course of occupational therapy and reviewed with Jill and her family prior to discharge.

Tips and Advice From the Field

Suitability for Practice

Occupational therapy work in an outpatient setting is a good fit for entry-level practitioners, especially those with experience gained during their clinical affiliations. Outpatient rehabilitation offers the opportunity to work within a department, as well as with an interdisciplinary team, which can provide consistency and mentorship.

When selecting an outpatient facility, it is important to inquire about the supervision and training available upon starting a new position, including observation hours (e.g., for treatment sessions or evaluations) or training on documentation (e.g., for the electronic medical records system). In an outpatient setting, new graduates typically have criteria to meet to demonstrate their knowledge under a senior or supervising therapist. Competency assessments allow for support during the transition to independent practice, as well as allow a facility to determine a clinician's comprehension and readiness.

New graduates should pursue a field of interest that allows them to be provided with proper mentorship to meet their professional goals, whether it is learning under a CHT, a vision and vestibular-certified clinician, or a clinician certified in modality use. More generalized outpatient settings can allow for more diverse learning in the orthopedic realm before pursuing a specialty.

New graduates starting their occupational therapy career in an outpatient setting should learn the facility's specifications and typical diagnoses seen, which will help guide the type of materials to be incorporated into a personal review to maximize their success when entering practice. For example, reviewing ROM, MMT, and safe body mechanics will allow for their proper and accurate implementation. If edema is a common patient impairment, practitioners would review utilizing a volumeter, circumferential measurements, figure 8 measurements, and recording pitting severity. Reviewing the MAS as a measurement of spasticity may be handy for a facility that treats patients with neurodevelopmental disabilities such as cerebral palsy.

Many qualities factor into determining employment suitability for outpatient practice. In outpatient rehabilitation, clinicians see only a snapshot of what is occurring in a patient's day-to-day life. Therefore, a clinician in this setting must have strong communication skills to obtain a detailed and descriptive picture of a patient's personal experiences to supplement objective measures. Communication skills in this setting extend to education on strategies and HEPs to ensure proper and safe intervention implementation.

In outpatient practice, occupational therapy clinicians typically work with patients on a consistent basis. Therefore, the ability to establish positive therapeutic rapport is central to optimizing patient outcomes. This rapport allows for honest and open conversations between patients and clinicians about their main concerns and how they are manifesting in their everyday tasks. Therapists in this setting should be open-minded to issues of diversity so that they are implementing treatment that meets a patient's functional and culturally relevant concerns (Agner, 2020).

Occupational therapists in outpatient practice must be flexible and adaptable. Scheduling may change due to cancellations and the ongoing evaluations scheduled. In addition, intervention planning is a significant part of the occupational therapy process. In outpatient practice, clinicians may not have all of the updated patient information on functional and medical status from nurses or aides. In turn, the ability to adjust treatment based on patient needs or new symptomatology since their previous visit is crucial to maximizing care.

Initiative is an important quality in an outpatient setting. Interdisciplinary practice is important, whether it is communicating with the client's primary care physician, specialist, or social worker, because a patient's outpatient resources may extend beyond a specific facility. Thus, it is essential to have a proper continuum of care with all required health information, and occupational therapists may need to seek out this information. In addition, because technology, treatment modalities, and methods are always changing, the abilities to evolve and utilize all available resources are important when developing clinical expertise.

Continuing Education and Resources

New graduates should ask questions. To understand previously known or new information, one must comprehend the patient population's needs and individual patients' specific areas of concern. Learning from textbooks and educators that began in the classroom provides the groundwork for entry-level practitioners. Using the textbooks and resources from academic institutions is crucial to maintaining that foundational knowledge. Once entering clinical practice, continuing education is necessary. Pursuing courses on skills that can be further strengthened or on topics of interest that are relevant to practice is important. For example, AOTA offers various resources, including access to research articles and current news and events, as well as information on continuing education courses around the nation (AOTA, 2022).

The goal of all patients seen on an outpatient level is to address performance capacity deficits that are impacting function at home, work, and in the community. Patients are typically residing in their most natural context and reintegrating into their daily occupations. Using the information provided from patients' daily experiences is imperative to maximize safety and function to support engagement. The objective measurements and subjective reports can guide treatment. Patients choose to seek out occupational therapy services; therefore, it is important to set relevant and realistic intervention goals by working collaboratively with them, thus motivating them for treatment.

References

Agner, J. (2020). Moving from cultural competence to cultural humility in occupational therapy: A paradigm shift. *The American Journal of Occupational Therapy, 74*(4), 7404347010p1–7404347010p7. https://doi.org/10.5014/ajot.2020.038067

American Occupational Therapy Association. (2017). *Acute-care.* Author.

American Occupational Therapy Association. (2022). *Continuing education and professional development.* https://www.aota.org/Education-Careers/Continuing-Education.aspx?gclid=EAIaIQobChMIzKnT2sey9QIVEPjICho1bw71EAAYAiAAEgISyvD_BwE

American Speech-Language-Hearing Association. (2006). *The Functional Independence Measure.* Author.

Beebe, J. A., & Lang, C. E. (2009). Relationships and responsiveness of six upper extremity function tests during the first six months of recovery after stroke. *Journal of Neurologic Physical Therapy, 33*(2), 96–103. https://doi.org/10.1097/NPT.0b013e3181a33638

Bohannon, R. W., & Smith, M. B. (1987). Interrater reliability of a modified ashworth scale of muscle spasticity. *Physical Therapy, 67*, 206–207. https://doi.org/10.1093/ptj/67.2.206

Centers for Medicare & Medicaid Services. (2012). *Clarifications for the IRF coverage requirements.* https://www.cms.gov/Medicare/Medicare-Fee-for-Service-Payment/InpatientRehabFacPPS/Downloads/Complete-List-of-IRF-Clarifications-Final-Document.pdf

Centers for Medicare & Medicaid Services. (2018). *IRF medical coverage requirements.* ttps://www.cms.gov/outreach-and-education/medicare-learning-network-mln/mlnmattersarticles

Flinn, N., Trombly-Latham, C., & Podolski, C. (2008). Assessing abilities and capacities in: Range of motion, strength, and endurance. In M. V. Radomski & C. A. Trombly-Latham (Eds.), *Occupational therapy for physical dysfunction* (6th ed., pp. 91–185). Williams & Wilkins.

Gauthier, L., Dehaut, F., & Joanette, Y. (1989). The Bells Test: a quantitative and qualitative test for visual neglect. *International Journal of Clinical Neuropsychology, 11*, 49-54.

Gladstone, D. J., Danells, C. J., & Black, S. E. (2002). The Fugl-Meyer Assessment of motor recovery after stroke: A critical review of its measurement properties. *Neurorehabilitation and neural repair, 16*(3), 232–240.

Harb, A., & Kishner, S. (2022). Modified Ashworth Scale. *StatPearls.* https://www.ncbi.nlm.nih.gov/books/NBK554572/

Inouye, S. (1988). *The Confusion Assessment Method.* NCBI.

Jette, A., Haley S. M., & Coster, W. (2017). *The Boston University Activity Measure for Post Acute Care.* Pearson. https://www.pearsonassessments.com/store/usassessments/en/Store/Professional-Assessments/Cognition-%26-Neuro/Activity-Measure-for-Post-Acute-Care/p/P100003000.html

Katz, N., Itzkovich, M., Averbuch, S., & Elazar, B. (2002). The Loewenstein Occupational Therapy Cognitive Assessment (LOTCA) battery for brain-injured patients: Reliability and validity. *American Journal of Occupational Therapy, 83*, 1179.

Keith, R. A., Granger, C. V., Hamilton, B. B., & Sherwin, F. S. (1987). The Functional Independence Measure: A new tool for rehabilitation. In M. G. Eisenberg & R. C. Grzesiak (Eds.), *Advances in clinical rehabilitation* (pp. 6–18). Springer.

Lang, C. E., Bland, M. D., Bailey, R. R., Schaefer, S. Y., & Birkenmeier, R. L. (2013). Assessment of upper extremity impairment, function, and activity following stroke: Foundations for clinical decision making. *Journal of Hand Therapy, 26*(2), 104–115. https://doi.org/10.1016/j.jht.2012.06.005

Mathiowetz, V., Volland, G., Kashman, N., & Weber, K. (1985a). Adult norms for the Box and Block Test of manual dexterity. *American Journal of Occupational Therapy, 39*(6), 386–391. https://doi.org/10.5014/ajot.39.6.386

Mathiowetz, V., Weber, K., Kashman, N., & Volland, G. (1985b). Adult norms for the 9-Hole Peg Test of finger dexterity. *Occupational Therapy Journal of Research, 5*(1), 24–38.

Menon, A., & Korner-Bitensky, N. (2004). Evaluating unilateral spatial neglect post stroke: Working your way through the maze of assessment choices. *Top Stroke Rehabilitation, 11*(3), 41-66.

Nasreddine, Z. S., Phillips, N. A., Bédirian, V., Charbonneau, S., Whitehead, V., Collin, I., Cummings, J. L., & Chertkow, H. (2005). The Montreal Cognitive Assessment, MoCA: A brief screening tool for mild cognitive impairment. *Journal of American Geriatrics Society, 53*(4), 695-6999. https://doi.org/10.1111/j.1532-5415.2005.53221.x

Roberts, T. T., Leonard, G. R., & Cepela, D. J. (2017). Classifications in brief: American Spinal Injury Association (ASIA) impairment scale. *Clinical Orthopaedics and Related Research, 475*(5), 1499-1504. https://doi.org/10.1007/s11999-016-5133-4.

Rogers, A. T., Bai, G., Lavin, R. A., & Anderson, G. F. (2016). Higher hospital spending on occupational therapy is associated with lower readmission rates. *Medical Care Research Revision, 74*(6), 668-686. https://doi.org/10.1177/1077558716666981a

Toglia, J. P. (1993). *Contextual Memory Test*. Therapy Skill Builders.

Vanbellingen, T., Kersten, B., Van Hemelrijk, B., Van de Winckel, A., Bertschi, M., Müri, R., De Weerdt, W., & Bohlhalter, S. (2010). Comprehensive assessment of gesture production: A new test of upper limb apraxia (TULIA). *European Journal of Neurology, 17*(1), 59-66. https://doi.org/10.1111/j.1468-1331.2009.02741.x

Whyte, J., Hart, T., Bode, R. K., Malec, J. F. (2003). The Moss Attention Rating Scale for traumatic brain injury: Initial psychometric assessment. *Archives of Physical Medicine and Rehabilitation, 84*(2), 268-276.

Wilson, B. A., Alderman, N., Burgess, P. W., Emslie, H., & Evans, J. J. (1996). *Behavioural assessment of the dysexecutive syndrome*. Harcourt Assessment.

2

Pediatric Sensory Gym

Esty Spitzer, OTD, OTR/L

Pediatric Sensory Gym in a Nutshell

The pediatric sensory gym is an outpatient pediatric occupational therapy clinic. Children with various diagnoses or developmental delays (DDs) receive occupational therapy services to help them function optimally in their environment. Ages and diagnoses typically can vary and include but are not limited to attention-deficit/hyperactivity disorder, cerebral palsy, autism spectrum disorder, sensory-processing disorder, seizure disorders, and DDs.

Some children who receive occupational therapy services at a sensory gym may receive their education in a typical classroom but require additional related services to function well in that classroom, in social settings, and with family members and peers. Treatment sessions usually are funded by the Department of Education, Department of Health for Early Intervention, private insurance, or private pay. Most students attend therapy after school hours or during the weekends; however, some parents may choose to pull their child out of school during the school day for therapy.

A variety of treatment frameworks can be used at a sensory gym. This chapter focuses on evaluation and the sensory integration frame of reference, reflex integration techniques, vestibular rehabilitation, and neurorehabilitation interventions.

Discharge planning for children receiving services in a sensory gym is a process that the parents or caregiver, the child, and the therapist are all part of. They discuss the different options for transitioning services. The therapist makes various suggestions to the parents based on the child's current level of function. These suggestions can include a home program as well as beneficial equipment for the child. For example, the therapist may recommend implementing a sensory diet at home and

Akselrud, R. (Ed.). *Quintessential Occupational Therapy:*
A Guide to Areas of Practice (pp 15-19).
© 2023 Taylor & Francis Group.

having equipment, such as a weighted vest. It is important for the therapist to train the caregiver in sensory stimulation or inhibition for the child, such as proprioception or vestibular input. The main goal of the process is to promote optimal daily function for the child (American Occupational Therapy Association, 2020).

Evaluation and Assessments

Children who receive occupational therapy services at a sensory gym often have sensory-processing difficulties, which can manifest as an array of deficits. When meeting a child and caregiver for the first time, occupational therapists participate in a comprehensive intake that includes questioning caregivers to determine any DDs or diagnoses that are of concern. The assessment includes a discussion about a child's developmental milestones, birth and medical history, past and current therapies, and difficulties and strengths. One standardized assessment, the Sensory Profile 2 (SP–2), developed by Winnie Dunn, PhD, OTR, FAOTA, can help determine a child's sensory challenges by placing scores on a continuum from the mean to standard deviations from the mean (Dunn, 2014).

In addition, a discussion with caregivers includes inquiring about their child's sensory-processing difficulties. Determining a child's registration or arousal levels, seeking or avoiding tendencies, discrimination, and modulation abilities can help occupational therapists develop an individualized intervention plan and home exercise program (HEP) to help every child improve in their sensory-processing challenges. Other caregiver questions can include a child's eating habits, sleep patterns, defensive tendencies toward clothing or bathing, activities of daily living, tantrums, emotional states, anxiety, fears, "on-the-go" tendencies, safety awareness, awareness of self and others in space, transitioning abilities, and rigidity or flexibility tendencies.

Some children with sensory issues may have retained primitive reflexes. During an assessment, occupational therapists conduct manual reflex testing to see if the main reflexes that hinder success are integrated. On the basis of a combination of manual reflex testing, child presentation, and caregiver and professional reports, therapists can create a customized intervention plan and HEP to integrate these nonintegrated reflexes. This plan can consist of, for example, rhythmic movement training, targeted reflex integration exercises and isometric exercises, archetype movements, calming techniques, tactile integration protocols, mindfulness, and yoga.

These exercises are carried out during therapy sessions, as well as at home or school, for a minimum of five times per week. Caregivers, general education and special education itinerant teachers, other professionals, and siblings are often recruited to assist with the carry over to HEPs.

Some commonly used assessment tools include the following:

- The Peabody Developmental Motor Scales–Second Edition
- The Bruininks-Oseretsky Test of Motor Proficiency–Second Edition
- The SP–2
- The Tansley Standard Visual Figures Test
- Manual reflex testing

The Peabody Developmental Motor Scales–Second Edition (Folio & Fewell, 2000) evaluates gross and fine motor skills development. This assessment includes gross motor subtests (reflexes, stationary, locomotion, object manipulation) and fine motor subtests (grasping, visual–motor integration; Folio & Fewell, 2000).

The Bruininks-Oseretsky Test of Motor Proficiency–Second Edition is used to evaluate gross and fine motor skills (Bruininks & Bruininks, 2005). Four categories consist of two subtests per classification: fine motor precision, fine motor integration, manual dexterity, upper limb coordination, bilateral coordination, balance, running speed and agility, and strength.

The SP–2 evaluates sensory-processing patterns in the context of everyday life and identifies how these may be contributing to or interfering with participation at home and in school (Dunn, 2014). The form is completed by primary caregivers.

The Tansley Standard Visual Figures Test presents eight figures (circle, cross, square, X, triangle, upturned box, diamond, Union Jack) that are to be copied freehand to a blank piece of paper. This test assesses visual–perceptual skills (Blythe, 2005).

Manual reflex testing evaluates various developmental primitive reflexes and the strength of their presence in a child (Blythe, 2005). Some children may maintain almost all of their primitive reflexes, which are likely contributing to the sensory-seeking tendencies identified in the SP–2. Implementing a reflex-integrating intervention plan can benefit children as they continue to mature.

Interventions

Sensory Integration Framework

Sensory integration as defined by Dr. Anna Jean Ayres (1972) is "both a neurological process and a theory of the relationship between the neurological process and behavior. It is the neurological process that organizes sensation from one's own body and from the environment and makes it possible to use the body effectively within the environment" (p. 11). The main premises of sensory integration theory are as follows:

- The brain is plastic throughout life.
- Brain organization exists in a hierarchy.
- Sensory integration is focused in the brain stem.
- Treatment requires active participation using the just-right challenge.
- The central nervous system either seeks or avoids sensory information.
- All sensory information is processed and integrated to produce an adaptive response (Ayres, 1972).

Reflex Integration Framework

The *Reflex Integration Framework* can guide assessment and treatment. The life cycle of a reflex includes both the emerge and develop stages. In the emerge stage, during typical development, various types of stimulation or another reflex can trigger a new reflex to begin its life cycle (Story & Kane, 2013). Progress of a reflex depends on factors such as environment, task, experiences, and integration of the reflexes that came before it. In the develop stage, as a reflex is stimulated, its movement patterns are expressed (Story & Kane, 2013). This process repeats many times in the course of reflex development.

Providing stimulation to an infant is critical for reflex development. Some children who need occupational therapy services still have some of their primitive reflexes, and these can hinder their success in different areas of life (Story & Kane, 2013).

Integrating reflexes, which are the foundation of the nervous system, is crucial for learning skills. Incomplete integration of childhood reflexes can be mild to severe and can contribute to attention-deficit/hyperactivity disorder, anxiety, speech and learning disorders, DDs, difficulties with coordination, behavioral problems, depression, fatigue, lack of confidence, and poor self-esteem (Pecuch et al., 2021). Like a block tower, all later development depends on the support of this foundation.

Brain Gym and Neurolinks

Brain Gym, a quick way to activate a child's highest performance potential, helps reduce feelings of stress induced by *fight-or-flight* tendencies caused by the sympathetic nervous system (Equilibrium, 2020). In fight or flight, muscles contract, the body releases cholesterol, heart rate increases, pupils dilate, the digestive system shuts down, breathing becomes quick and shallow, and white blood cell count increases. Stress response symptoms include unlocking muscles and weakness, being prone to accidents, losing interest and procrastinating, and experiencing mental fogginess, dizziness, and fatigue (Dennison & Dennison, 1989). The Brain Gym uses simple movements to integrate the right and left sides of the brain for tasks.

Neurolinks Physio-Neuro Therapy (2015) helps a child learn to attend, focus, and sharpen their brain. These specific exercises help the brain mature and target different parts of the brain in order for children to keep up with the pace of the classroom and other settings (Neurolinks Physio-Neuro Therapy, 2015).

Wilbarger Techniques

The Wilbarger Deep Pressure and Proprioceptive Technique and Oral Tactile Technique, which previously was referred to as the Wilbarger Brushing Protocol, utilizes targeted sensory modulation techniques developed by Patricia Wilbarger, MEd, OTR, FAOTA (Wilbarger, 1984; Wilbarger & Wilbarger, 1991, 2002). Roy et al. (2018) suggest that the psychological well-being of an individual can be affected through the Wilbarger protocol and therapeutic holding as they are both effective tactile reconciliation treatments. The protocol for the Wilbarger includes brushing, joint pressure, and weight. The therapist applies pressure to different parts of the child's body, such as giving joint compressions. The therapist brushes the child's skin and then utilizes a substantial weight, such as a weighted blanket, as part of the treatment. The treatment is repeated every few hours for a few minutes. Studies indicate that deep touch pressure can be beneficial and have an effect on calming and improved control of behavior in children (Roy et al., 2018).

Tips and Advice From the Field

When treating children in a sensory gym, it is crucial for occupational therapists to stay focused on a child's goals and communicate these to caregivers. Sensory gyms can appear like typical indoor play spaces, and as such, therapists must be clear about children's goals and the clinical reasoning behind which pieces of equipment are used for treatment. Therapists must explain their rationale to caregivers so that they can also understand the reasoning behind the choices and thus can more successfully complete an HEP with a child.

One piece of equipment or toy can be used to reach a variety of goals for children of all ages. Occupational therapy's goal is to provide client-centered, evidence-based practice, and by planning and reflecting on treatment sessions, therapists are focusing on best practice.

References

American Occupational Therapy Association. (2020). Occupational therapy practice framework: Domain and process (4th ed.). *American Journal of Occupational Therapy, 74*(Suppl. 2), 7412410010p1-7412410010p87. https://doi.org/10.5014/ajot.2020.74S2001

Ayres, A. J. (1972). *Sensory integration and learning disorders.* Western Psychological Corporation.

Blythe, S. G. (2005). *Reflexes, learning, and behavior: A window into a child's mind.* Fern Ridge Press.

Bruininks, R. H., & Bruininks, B. D. (2005). Bruininks-Oseretsky Test of Motor Proficiency, Second Edition (BOT-2). *APA PsycTests.* https://doi.org/10.1037/t14991-000

Dennison, P. E., & Dennison, G. E. (1989). *Brain Gym: Teacher's edition.* Edu Kinesthetics.

Dunn, W. (2014). *Sensory Profile—2.* Pearson. https://pearsonclinical.in/solutions/sensory-profile-2/

Equilibrium. (2020). About Brain Gym. *Equilibrium Kinesiology and Brain Gym Supplies.* https://www.kinesiologyshop.com/about-us/

Folio, M. R., & Fewell, R. R. (2000). *PDMS-2: Peabody Developmental Motor Scales.* Pro-Ed.

Neurolinks Physio-Neuro Therapy. (2015). *How can Neurolinks help?* https://neurolinkstherapy.com/what-is-neurolinks/

Pecuch, A., Gieysztor, E., Wolanska, E., Telenga, M., & Paprocka-Borowicz, M. (2021). Primitive reflex activity in relation to motor skills in healthy preschool children. *Brain Sciences, 11*(8), 967. https://doi.org/10.3390/brainsci11080967

Roy, A., Ghosh, H., & Bhatt, I. (2018). A study on tactile defensiveness in children with autism spectrum disorder. *Journal of National Development, 31*(2), 75-83. https://doi.org/10.1044/2019ajslp-19-00045

Story, S., & Kane, S. (2013). *Brain and sensory foundations, neurodevelopmental movements for physical, emotional, social, and learning skills.* Moveplaythrive. https://www.moveplaythrive.com/44-class-descriptions/176-brain-and-sensory-foundations-first-level

Wilbarger, J., & Wilbarger, P. (2002). Wilbarger approach to treating sensory defensiveness and clinical application of the sensory diet. Sections in alternative and complementary programs for intervention. In A. C. Bundy, E. A. Murray, & S. Lane (Eds.), *Sensory integration: Theory and practice* (2nd ed.). F. A. Davis.

Wilbarger, P. (1984). Planning an adequate sensory diet—Application of sensory processing theory during the first year of life. *Zero to Three,* 7–12.

Wilbarger, P., & Wilbarger, J. (1991). *Sensory defensiveness in children aged 2–12: An intervention guide for parents and other caretakers.* Avanti Educational Programs.

3

Hand Therapy

James Battaglia, EdD, OTR/L, CHT
and April O'Connell, OT/L, CHT, ACSM

Hand Therapy in a Nutshell

Hand therapy is a practice area that provides great flexibility for occupational therapists who may wish to work per diem, part-time, full-time, or even overtime. Hand therapists treat a wide variety of diagnoses, with patient populations ranging from pediatrics to adults to geriatrics. The most frequent diagnoses include tendinitis of the wrist, elbow, or shoulder; carpal tunnel syndrome; trigger finger (stenosing tenosynovitis); osteoarthritis; ulnar neuropathy; distal radius and metacarpal fractures; and rotator cuff tears. Other diagnoses include finger or carpal fractures, rheumatoid arthritis or systemic disease affecting the upper extremity, Dupuytren's contracture, ganglion cysts, ligamentous injuries, radial head or neck fractures, and tendon repairs. Less frequent diagnoses include various pediatric conditions (unless one works in an exclusive pediatric facility), brachial plexus injury, neurological conditions, and wound care.

Evaluation and Assessments

Evaluations, completed during the first therapy session, provide occupational therapists with a chance to interview patients, understanding their medical history, functional demands, and deficits, as well as undertaking a complete systems review (see Appendix B). Therapists next examine the involved body part, looking at both extremities and the structures distal and proximal to the injured area. A detailed plan of care and functional, pertinent goals are then established and reviewed so that patients understand their prognosis and expectations. During this time, therapists can build rapport and seek patient "buy-in" to the therapy process.

Akselrud, R. (Ed.). *Quintessential Occupational Therapy:*
A Guide to Areas of Practice (pp 21-39).
© 2023 Taylor & Francis Group.

Evaluations range from 30 to 60 minutes. Assessments included in a hand therapy evaluation include but are not limited to goniometry for active range of motion (AROM) and passive range of motion (PROM) measurements, circumferential edema measurements, skin integrity and wound assessment, manual muscle testing, 9-Hole Peg and other dexterity tests, dynamometer grip strength testing, and pinch gauge testing. Sensory testing may include moving and static two-point discrimination, the Semmes–Weinstein Monofilament Test, temperature, proprioception, kinesthesia, and stereognosis.

A full battery of tests relevant to each diagnosis can be performed. Typically, these tests are used in a cluster for best specificity. For example, when testing patients presenting with lateral elbow pain, the test battery may include Cozen's Test (resisted wrist extension), the Long Finger Test, Tinel's Test over the radial nerve, and the Varus Elbow Stability Test. Occupational therapists also assess extension, flexion, supination, and pronation range of motion (ROM) at the elbow and forearm, as well as shoulder and wrist ROM. Pain with palpation is noted. These tests can help provide a reliable rationale for patients' pain and give clinicians a starting point for developing an intervention plan.

In addition, several patient-rated outcome measures have been validated for upper extremity diagnoses. The most commonly used are the Upper Extremity Functional Index and the Disabilities of the Arm, Shoulder, and Hand Questionnaire, as well as the Quick Disabilities of the Arm, Shoulder, and Hand (Hudak et al., 1996). The visual analog scale is also a well-accepted way to rate patient pain. Patient-rated outcome measures should be given every 5 to 10 visits, and the visual analog scale should be asked at every treatment session so that clinicians can ascertain if their intervention is helping patients reach their goals (Delgado et al., 2018). Employment interviews conducted in a hand therapy setting may not always seek to determine which candidate knows the most about upper extremity conditions. Anyone can read a protocol book; employers want to know more how a therapist might handle difficult patient situations and how well candidates can think quickly "on their feet." Some sample interview questions might include the following:

You are evaluating Mrs. B, who is a 72-year-old right-hand dominant woman 4 weeks postoperation from a distal radius fracture status post open reduction internal fixation (DRFx s/p ORIF). She has just had her cast removed and needs an orthosis fabricated for her as well as an evaluation. Her Rx states, "R DRFx s/p ORIF. A/AAROM and light activity. Orthosis fabrication for when out and sleeping."

Mrs. B is expressing a lot of fear about moving her hand and reinjuring it. She states that she takes care of her husband, who is 75 years old and does not move around well. She also likes cooking and shopping.

- *Question 1: What type of orthosis would you fabricate for the patient?*
- *Question 2: What would be your plan of care?*
- *Question 3: How might you address her fear to move her hand? How might this impact your therapy and her outcome?*
- *Question 4: What types of therapeutic exercises would you provide, and how would this tie into your written patient goals?*
- *Question 5: What types of resources might you provide to assist the patient with taking care of her husband, as well as help her with cooking while she is beginning therapy?*

In this interview, the employer is looking to not only determine if candidates know a basic treatment plan for a common diagnosis but also how they would elicit patient buy-in to the therapy process. How could they convince the patient to trust that they are there to help them reach their goals and not to hurt them? How could they factor in the patient's own motivation to get better to take care of her husband? What resources might they utilize (e.g., social work, meal delivery services) while Mrs. B works toward increased use of her hand? Creative thinking as well as always focusing on patient-centered rehabilitation goals is a trait of good hand therapists.

Interventions

Many diagnosis-specific treatment protocols are available to hand therapists, and hand therapy literature is always evolving to reflect the best evidence-based practices. Occupational therapists working in hand therapy, however, must also understand each patient's unique nature. Therapists of all experience levels must be aware of their own individual practice routines and habits to avoid falling into the *one-size-fits-all* mindset. Therefore, therapists must have several tools in their therapy "tool belt" to offer patients. Therapists must ensure that treatment modalities and techniques are always used appropriately based on an individual patient's needs in combination with supportive evidence.

The length of therapy sessions varies by clinic and often reflects the type of health insurance reimbursement the clinic receives. Many clinics schedule patients for 30-minute treatment sessions and dovetail sessions as patients independently finish their previously instructed therapeutic exercises. Some clinics accepting a variety of in- and out-of-network health insurance can schedule up to four patients an hour (in 15-minute blocks) with overlapping treatment sessions. For example, a therapist might give 15 minutes of hands-on manual therapy and then alternate with the next patient, who may be provided with a heat modality or be placed on the upper body ergometer as they "warm up," while the first patient is instructed in therapeutic exercise. In this clinic, 20 to 25 patients may be seen in 1 day. On certain days when associated physicians have office hours, walk-in orthosis fabrication appointments must also be accommodated. Some clinics will employ a certified occupational therapy assistant to help facilitate patient care in busier settings. A certified occupational therapy assistant implements and documents occupational therapist interventions while reporting back to the occupational therapist about clients' progress (National Board for Certification in Occupational Therapy, 2022). In clinics that accept only out-of-network insurance or private payment, therapists may see patients one-on-one for up to 1 hour, seeing six to eight patients in 1 day.

All patients require a comprehensive note to be written after treatment to reflect their pain level, their subjective report on their current status, what occurred during treatment, the therapist's assessment of their progress toward their predetermined goals, and plan for their next session. Patient-rated outcome measures should be administered every 5 to 10 visits to track a patient's progress throughout therapy. Patient-rated outcome measures are often required to be submitted when asking for additional therapy sessions from insurance companies and are a good assessment of a patient's subjective account of their functional status. Notes should always be accurate and detailed in order to be reimbursed for the treatment performed and reflect what is billed to a patient's health insurance.

Patient notes are also part of the legal medical record and can be used in court. However, note writing time may not be included in a therapist's daily work schedule.

Discharge Planning

Discharge planning in outpatient hand rehabilitation is a collaborative effort between the patient and therapist. Understanding the functional needs of the patient, their commitment to continued participation in a home exercise program (HEP), and motivation to return to particular daily activities are all considered in this planning. First, the patient and therapist should engage in envisioning the discharge plan ahead of the final session, ideally at the initial evaluation. This will set the patient up in a positive manner to manage their expectations of what therapy will entail so that patients do not get blindsided that a discharge from therapy is looming unexpectedly. The patient's goals should be established early in the rehabilitation process and considered when formulating the treatment and discharge plan. When the goals set forth in therapy are achieved, patients should be prepared to transition to a home program and return to functional tasks. Though progress is never a guarantee, envisioning where the patient should be by the time they leave the therapist's care will help frame the discussion about how therapy will progress, and what the expectations are for when the patient is discharged from care. Once the patient has achieved the goals set forth in therapy (or gains have slowed and the patient is no longer in a restorative phase of rehabilitation), the therapist should have a discussion with the patient regarding the plan for discharge in the near future. On the discharge date, final measurements should be taken, a patient-rated functional outcome measure should be completed, and the patient should have their HEP reviewed and modified to meet their current level of function. Activity modification should also be reviewed if tasks remain a challenge for the patient. Patients often feel the need to extend therapy beyond this restorative phase so therapists need to prepare the patient ahead of their final session and be prepared to inform that patient of gains (or lack of gains) during the last assessment period. Once the final session is complete, a discharge note is written and forwarded to the referring physician to make them aware of the patient's status at discharge. It is often helpful to remind the patient that you are always available to answer any questions they may have in the future, and any reason they should return to the doctor for reevaluation. Having clear expectations and goals, a plan for treatment that envisions the status of the patient at discharge, and collaboration with the patient in preparation for discharge will assist in a smooth discontinuation of treatment. Understanding what the literature says in terms of outcomes for a particular diagnosis is also extremely helpful in order to guide the patient in what they may achieve, and then create a concrete plan for discharge that they can work on independently. The more the therapist can guide the patient as an active participant in their rehabilitation vs. having a passive approach, the better prepared your patient will be for discharge as they will feel empowered and independent.

In the instance that a patient is having other symptoms that may warrant further inspection, the hand therapist should be well equipped in knowing how to perform a screen and then referring out to the appropriate physician. For example, if a patient is still complaining of lateral elbow pain after several months of occupational therapy, and they have concomitant neck pain, a referral back to the physician to evaluate the neck would be appropriate.

Tips and Advice From the Field

Hand therapists should be well versed in all diagnoses, ranging from the fingertips to the shoulder girdle and brachial plexus. It is also important to understand cervical and thoracic conditions, how to screen for these, and when to refer to an appropriate specialist when deficits in function are identified. It is imperative that therapists have a good understanding of how the trunk and lower extremities function to transfer power to the upper extremities.

Postural defects, for example, can play a role in the prognosis and resolution of carpal tunnel syndrome (Erickson et al., 2019). Furthermore, a case series by Bhatt (2013) identified that strengthening of the lower and middle trapezius musculature helped decrease patient pain scores and increase grip strength in patients with lateral epicondylalgia. Therefore, it is beneficial for hand therapists to seek continuing education courses that examine the entire body to avoid falling into a limited scope of treatment.

Occupational therapists new to hand therapy should review protocols provided by the referring physician if available, as well as the level of evidence within the treatment approach, including relevant clinical practice guidelines (American Academy of Orthopaedic Surgeons, 2016) and systematic reviews. Not only will this literature review help novice therapists gain a better understanding of how to build an algorithm for a patient's intervention but also can guide them in using empirically supported interventions.

A typical day in hand therapy practice can be busy. Therapists often juggle scheduled patients along with walk-in patients requiring orthotic fabrication after having a cast removed by their physician. Hand therapy is ideal for new graduates who are willing to take the initiative to attend basic continuing education courses and be motivated to research patient conditions, treatment techniques, and protocols. Furthermore, new graduates should have had at least one Level II fieldwork in hand therapy. Therapists pursuing a career in hand therapy might consider applying for a position in a hospital or clinic that offers shadowing or mentoring opportunities. Prospective hand therapists must be willing to ask many questions of their supervisors or mentors, accept and process feedback, and proactively review the literature independent of work hours.

The certified hand therapist (CHT) designation is provided by the Hand Therapy Certification Commission (HTCC). To obtain this designation, therapists must be occupational or physical therapists in good standing, complete a minimum of 3 years of certified or licensed practice, complete a minimum of 4,000 hours of direct practice experience in upper extremity rehabilitation, and pass the CHT examination (HTCC, 2019; for more information, see www.HTCC.org).

Hand therapists must understand each patient's values and the occupations in which they engage. It can be surprising what daily activities patients value, and therapists might have different adaptations to offer some patients that they might not have considered.

Many great courses, books, blogs, and websites exist for occupational therapists who want to enter hand therapy practice. Appendix A is a brief list of some helpful resources. This list is not exhaustive, so therapists should also explore local opportunities for continuing education and resources.

Stories of Successes and Failures

Every occupational therapist's career is filled with successes and failures. Even the greatest therapists can tell of instances when they wished they had done something a bit differently with a patient. Success does not always come with a patient receiving full ROM or strength; sometimes success is the impact a therapist makes on a patient's long-term trajectory.

The following are experiences in the field:

A young girl from a local college, who had experienced a severe brachial plexopathy after a medical mishap during rotator cuff surgery, came into the clinic for hand therapy. The patient was a cheerleader who was very involved in cheerleading at her school and in the community. The patient had almost no function of her left upper extremity. She was quiet and a bit angry. She was mad that a physician had damaged her, was scared of what the future would hold, and did not see a bright path for her moving into adulthood. Cheerleading was the patient's life, and she had planned to work in the sport as a career. She also asked, "How am I going to be a mother?"

In the first few sessions, not much happened physically with this patient, but she had a renewed spirit and attitude about how she was going to pass this hurdle. It was in the therapist–patient relationship that the real work was being done—building rapport, establishing trust, and celebrating even the smallest victories—to prepare her for her future challenges. The therapist (J.B.) continued to treat her for many months and through many follow-up surgeries, making gains that built on each success. Slowly the patient's elbow started to move, then her wrist, and then her digits. Although full return of her hand function never happened, she was prepared to face these challenges through adaptation and perseverance. The therapist kept in touch with this patient over the years, who is now a mother of three children, working (although not in the field of cheerleading), and has many days of smiles rather than tears, fear, and anger. The success was not in her moving her arm but in the impact that therapy has made on her life (Bowering et al., 2013).

Failures and second guesses also can happen at any point in one's career. Although few of these failures are catastrophic, they do make one think about how to approach treatment. Occupational therapists will never stop learning about their own strengths and weaknesses as therapists.

Another experience noted from a therapist (J.B.) was a patient encountered for the first time who had complex regional pain syndrome (CRPS). The patient had had the condition for a while, which had developed after a fall on the stage resulting in an ankle injury. She was a professional singer who was unable to practice her craft because of pain in her lower extremity.

A few years after ankle surgery, the patient had begun to develop a change in sensation and pain in the left upper extremity and was referred to the therapist to address the possible development of CRPS in that extremity.

By this time, the therapist had been working for many years and had treated multiple patients with CRPS, which in some ways had clouded his better judgment when dealing with this particular patient. The therapist was fully prepared to convince her that she needed to address this condition head on by making changes in her daily routine and agreeing that mentally she was prepared to face her condition and overcome it. However, in this case, the therapist probably pressed harder, not physically but emotionally and mentally, than he should have. As a result, the patient shut down and pushed back against his ideas in their first session. She became angry and ambivalent toward treatment. The therapist had felt at the time that if they worked together to address her upper extremity symptoms (which may or may not have been CRPS), her condition would improve.

The patient, however, was not ready for that challenge. Thus, only one session was done with the therapist, and an important lesson was learned. Had the therapist met the patient at the place where she was early in the intervention, perhaps over time she would have been ready to address her condition in the way that the therapist had planned originally.

It is not certain that working differently would have led to a different outcome. For the future, the therapist will be more mindful in treatments with patients moving forward and learn from this experience.

Collaboration With Other Disciplines

Occupational therapists in hand therapy have ample opportunities to work together with other team members and disciplines to reach the optimal outcome for patients. Because CHTs can be either occupational or physical therapists, occupational therapists might work alongside physical therapists when treating patients, even though far more occupational than physical therapists work in hand therapy.

In an outpatient clinic, occupational therapists might share patients with physical therapists working on the hand or another body part. For example, in the case of an older patient who has fallen at home and is experiencing both hip and wrist fractures, it is likely that a physical therapist would work on recovery of hip motion and strength while working on ambulation, and an occupational therapist would treat the after effects of the distal radius fracture.

Occupational therapists might also work closely with a single or multiple hand surgeons in a hand therapy practice, along with associated physician assistants. Therefore, it is imperative that therapists maintain open lines of communication with surgeons and their team to ensure the best patient care. Surgeons may have specific postoperative protocols they prefer therapists to follow with their patients, so having a good understanding of the procedure, protocol, and follow-up required by a physician is important. Other disciplines that therapists may work with include nurses, nutritionists, physiatrists, exercise physiologists, and speech-language pathologists.

Therapists who are a good fit for hand therapy have several important qualities and strengths. First and foremost, therapists should have strong interpersonal skills and the ability to communicate effectively with patients, physicians, other health professionals, and patients' family members. Because hand therapists literally work hand-in-hand with patients, building rapport and listening to and understanding a patient's narratives, goals, and challenges, as well as the social and emotional challenges presented by hand injuries, is required. This rapport can affect the patient's ability to follow an HEP and can help determine how they are tolerating therapy.

Therapists also must have confidence in their ability to communicate with physicians and surgeons regarding a patient's condition and needs. It can be intimidating to call a surgeon's office to ask questions or request prescriptions for orthotic fabrication or other patient orders. Maintaining a good relationship with health providers will keep patients coming to the clinic, help maintain a referral base, and maximize patient outcomes.

Therapists working in hand therapy must be inquisitive and self-directed in their learning to develop in this practice area. Although therapists might treat the same limited number of conditions for the majority of the time, they will encounter diagnoses, surgical techniques, or protocols with which they are unfamiliar and thus will need to quickly familiarize themselves with these without time for extensive research. Being a self-directed, lifelong learner is essential to keep informed of new techniques, treatments, and protocols and will help prepare therapists for unforeseen circumstances.

Furthermore, therapists should have a thorough understanding of anatomy and upper extremity kinematics, and how they affect motion and lead to function. The upper extremity is a well-balanced machine. Identifying where imbalances occur in this system can make a difference in patient outcomes.

In addition, occupational therapists working in hand therapy must also have strong clinical reasoning skills. Although protocols exist that dictate the "typical" course of treatment, hand therapists are often tasked to see "the big picture" and adjust therapy sessions on the basis of patient status. For example, therapists might speed up or slow down a patient protocol based on the amount of scar tissue and limitation in joint mobility seen during a session. These actions require therapists to not only understand a patient's protocol, stages of healing, and precautions but also if patients are not responding in a "typical" fashion. Clinical reasoning and decision making must consider a patient's life context, how an injury can affect their daily life, and their daily occupational requirements.

Superior time management and organizational skills are necessary to successfully work in hand therapy. Occupational therapists often work in fast-paced environments with tight schedules and large numbers of patients. Therapists must often adjust to patients arriving outside of the scheduled time, accommodate walk-in patients, and be aware of the status of multiple patients working on exercise programs simultaneously, all while finding time to complete required daily documentation, insurance forms, and facility-required documents and tracking sheets. Without strong organizational and time management skills, therapists may fall behind and spend extended hours completing their daily work requirements.

Therapists must also be flexible in terms of work hours and days worked. Most hand therapy clinics attempt to accommodate early and late hour appointments. Therapists may work early morning and late night hours and on weekends. Therapists with limited time management skills might work more hours than anticipated to keep up with documentation requirements.

Suitability for Practice

Hand therapy can be a challenging but rewarding practice area. The following are a few tips for occupational therapy students and new clinicians:

- Students can discuss their interests with their academic fieldwork coordinator to obtain a Level II fieldwork placement in hand therapy practice, such as in a hand therapy clinic, a hospital, or another setting with a hand therapy department. Another therapist (J.B.) encounter at a Level II fieldwork at Bellevue Hospital Center in New York included splitting time between the inpatient rehabilitation unit and the hand clinic, and so the therapist experienced carrying a caseload in both areas of practice, working on their treatment and splinting skills under the supervision of a skilled occupational therapist CHT.
- Some schools offer a third "specialty" rotation in hand therapy. The 3 months of study required will not put students far behind their cohort, and they will have gained significant experience for their résumés.
- Our recommendations are the same for new graduates without hand therapy experience. Whereas it is difficult for new graduates without this experience to obtain a position in a private hand therapy clinic immediately out of school, working in the local medical center can provide exposure to hand therapy and may allow therapists to rotate through these areas.
- New graduates who are employed in outpatient hand therapy clinics must receive proper supervision. Inexperienced therapists cannot manage a full caseload alone with no one to ask

for clinical advice. Moreover, whether it be another therapist, a professor, or a physician, new therapists need a mentor to seek advice when stumped about a diagnosis or to help explain why a patient is not responding as anticipated. Mentors can provide insight gained from experience that a new therapist does not have yet.

- Great fellowship opportunities exist for new occupational therapists interested in specializing in hand rehabilitation. Fellowships provide an immersive hand therapy experience that prepares therapists to work with a wide range of hand therapy patients (for more information, visit https://www.htcc.org/continuing-education/fellowships).

- Because the CHT exam is comprehensive and challenging, it is important to begin preparing well in advance of the test date. Make a month-by-month plan of how to approach the material, leaving time to review areas that are challenging. Therapists cannot rely solely on practice hours to provide enough background to pass the exam. Finding a study partner with whom to practice questions or a mentor or coworker to regularly challenge and test knowledge is helpful.

- Therapists taking the CHT exam should keep a log of their treatment time. Noting the date, diagnosis, and treatment time will help create the record needed for the exam's application. Employers must verify therapists' work hours, and this record also can show supervisors what work has been done over a particular period of time.

- Because it is nearly impossible to teach all one needs to know about hand therapy in the few classes taught in school on this topic, it is important for occupational therapists to take continuing education courses, especially if paid by an employer.

- Occupational therapists learning how to fabricate custom orthoses must practice. Saving the scraps or small pieces of material left from another splint, heating them, seeing how they react to the heat and molding, and then applying them on a coworker, can show how the material reacts to heating, how it drapes, how much it can be manipulated before it cools, and how it conforms to a "patient." Practicing on a coworker is preferred to figuring out how the material works on an actual patient.

- Because therapists will be working "hand-in-hand" with patients over several months, it is important to build rapport. Engaging patients and building a relationship on the basis of trust and mutual respect requires therapists to be good listeners. Sometimes what patients say provides more information about their condition than does testing.

For information regarding continuing education courses, books, blogs, and websites about hand therapy, see Appendix A. Forms are in Appendices B and C.

References

American Academy of Orthopaedic Surgeons. (2016). *Management of carpal tunnel syndrome evidence-based clinical practice guideline.* https://www.aaos.org/quality/quality-programs/upper-extremity-programs/carpal-tunnel-syndrome/

Bhatt, J. B., Glaser, R., Chavez, A., & Yung, E. (2013). Middle and lower trapezius strengthening for the management of lateral epicondylalgia: A case report. *Journal of Orthopaedic and Sports Physical Therapy, 43*(11), 841-847. https://doi.org/10.2519/jospt.2013.4659

Bowering, K. J., O'Connell, N. E., Tabor, A., Catley, M. J., Leake, H. B., Moseley, G. L., & Stanton, T. R. (2013). The effects of graded motor imagery and its components on chronic pain: A systematic review and meta-analysis. *Journal of Pain, 14*(1), 3–13. https://doi.org/10.1016/j.jpain.2012.09.007

Delgado, D. A., Lambert, B. S., Boutris, N., McCulloch, P. C., Robbins, A. B., Moreno, M. R., & Harris, J. D. (2018). Validation of digital visual analog scale pain scoring with a traditional paper-based visual analog scale in adults. *Journal of the Academy of Orthopaedic Surgeons Global Research and Reviews, 2*(3), e088. https://doi.org/10.5435/JAAOSGlobal-D-17-00088

Erickson, M., Lawrence, M., Stegink Jansen, C. W., Coker, D., Amadio, P., Cleary, C., Altman, R., Beattie, P., Boeglin, E., Dewitt, J., Detullio, L., Ferland, A., Hughes, C., Kaplan, S., Killoran, D., Maitland, M. E., Mehta, S., Torburn, L., & Yung, E. (2019). Hand pain and sensory deficits: Carpal tunnel syndrome. *Journal of Orthopaedic and Sports Physical Therapy, 49*(5), CPG1–CPG85. https://doi.org/10.2519/jospt.2019.0301

Hand Therapy Certification Commission. (2019). *Salary survey results*. https://www.htcc.org/htcc/salary-survey-results

Hudak, P. L., Amadio, P. C., & Bombardier, C. (1996). Development of an upper extremity outcome measure: the DASH (disabilities of the arm, shoulder and hand) [corrected]. The Upper Extremity Collaborative Group (UECG). *American Journal of Industrial Medicine, 29*(6), 602-608. https://doi.org/10.1002/(SICI)1097-0274(199606)29:6<602::AID-AJIM4>3.0.CO;2-L

National Board for Certification in Occupational Therapy. (2022). *What does it mean to be a certified NBCOT?* https://www.nbcot.org/occupational-therapy/what-is-an-otr-or-cota

Appendix A: Continuing Education Courses, Books, Blogs, and Websites

There are many great courses, books, blogs, and websites out there for the therapist looking to enter hand therapy. Here is a brief list of some resources you might find helpful in your journey. By no means is this an exhaustive list of resources, so make sure you explore local opportunities for continuing education and resources.

Continuing Education Courses

- American Society of Hand Therapists (ASHT) Hand Therapy Review Course: Given in multiple locations, provides a comprehensive review of hand therapy topics including clinical reasoning, case discussion, and evidence-based practice. This course also offers a structured study approach when preparing for the CHT exam and can help to identify areas of strength and weakness prior to the exam. It is highly recommended you take this course prior to sitting for the CHT exam. See https://asht.org/.
- ASHT Hands-On Orthotics Workshop: Multiple locations and dates. Provides a hands-on experience for therapists looking to improve their splinting skills. See https://asht.org/.
- ASHT Live Webinars: ASHT also offers a wide range of webinars throughout the year on various topics related to hand therapy. See https://asht.org/.
- The HTCC provided an extensive list of regional courses related specifically to upper extremity rehabilitation. Visit the HTCC website at https://www.htcc.org/continuing-education.
- Doctors Demystify: Courses are provided by local surgeons covering various diagnoses of the upper extremity. Self-study courses are also available at the website (http://www.doctorsdemystify.com/product-category/live-courses/).
- Occupationaltherapy.com: Provides a range of online upper extremity rehabilitation courses for a yearly membership to the site. Currently $99.
- RehabEd.com: Provides live and online continuing education related to occupational therapy and with a focus on hand and upper extremity rehabilitation.
- Handtherapy.com: Provides a number of resources for the hand therapist, as well as online continuing education courses provided through liveconferences.com.
- Handlab.com: Online courses and DVD modules with a focus on hand rehabilitation provided by Judy Colditz, OT/L, CHT, FAOTA.

Books/Texts

- Skirven, T. M., Osterman, A. L., Fedorczyk, J., & Amadio, P. C. (2011). *Rehabilitation of the hand and upper extremity* (6th ed.). Mosby.
  - An indispensable text for any therapist working in the area of hand therapy. Recommended first purchase and study guide for the CHT exam!
- Weiss, S., & Rogers, L. (2019). *Hand and upper extremity rehabilitation: A quick reference guide and review* (4th ed.). Exploring Hand Therapy.
  - This is also a great resource for those studying for the CHT exam. Provides review of each topic with multiple choice questions and rationale for the answers.
- Iannotti, J. P., & Parker, R. D. (2013). *The Netter collection of medical illustrations: Musculoskeletal system: Part I upper limb* (2nd ed., Vol. 6). Elsevier Saunders.
- Neumann, D. A. (2017). *Kinesiology of the musculoskeletal system: Foundations of rehaabilitation* (3rd ed.). Elsevier.

- ○ Great text for understanding movement and function of the upper extremity.
- Kendall, F. P., McCreary, E. K., Provance, P. G., Rodgers, M. M., & Romani, W. A. (2005). *Muscles: Testing and function with posture and pain* (5th ed.). Lippincott Williams and Wilkins.
  - ○ Text provides in-depth explanation of manual muscle testing of the upper extremity.
- Cleland J., Koppenhaver, S., & Su, J. (2016). *Netter's orthopaedic clinical examination: An evidence-based approach* (3rd ed.). Elsevier.
- Bracciano, A. G. (2022). *Physical agent modalities: Theory and application for the occupational therapist* (3rd ed.). SLACK Incorporated.
- Coppard, B. M., & Lohman, H. (2015). *Introduction to orthotics: A clinical reasoning and problem-solving approach* (5th ed.). Mosby.
- Biel, A. (2019). *Trail guide to the body: A hands-on approach to locating muscles, bones, and more* (6th ed.). Books of Discovery.
- American Society of Hand Therapists. (2015). *Clinical assessment recommendations*. J. MacDermid, Ed. (3rd ed.).

Blogs, Websites, and Apps

- MyOTspot.com/blog/
- OTPotential.com
- WebPT.com/blog
- ASHT.org
- ASSH.org
- HTCC.org
- AOTA.org
- TheOThub.com
- Advance for Occupational Therapy Practitioners
- CORE Hand app
- Hand and Wrist Pro III app
- MoTrack Therapy app

Appendix B: Hand Therapy Initial Evaluation

Patient Name:	Date of Evaluation:
Date of Injury:	Rx Expires:
Date of Surgery:	60 Days From Start of Care:

Subjective Summary

Summary of relevant history:

Past medical and surgical history:

Precautions or contraindications:

Current medications:

Social history and work status:

Hand dominance:

Prior level of function:

Fall history:

Pain level/visual analog scale (0-10):

Pain location, frequency, and quality:

Patient goal:

Patient-rated outcome measure:

Objective Summary

Edema:

Circumferential edema measurement (in centimeters):

	WRIST CREASE	DISTAL PALMAR CREASE	PROXIMAL PHALANX
Left			
Right			

Skin integrity/scar quality:

Sensation:

Semmes–Weinstein Monofilament:

I	II	III	IV	V

Two-Point Discrimination:

I	II	III	IV	V

Range of motion:

JOINT	MOTION	AROM		PROM	
		Left	Right	Left	Right
Shoulder	Flexion				
	Extension				
	Abduction				
	External Rotation				
	Internal Rotation				
Elbow	Flexion				
	Extension				
Forearm	Pronation				
	Supination				
Wrist	Flexion				
	Extension				
	Ulnar Deviation				
	Radial Deviation				

HAND		AROM THUMB (I)	AROM INDEX (II)	AROM MIDDLE (III)	AROM RING (IV)	AROM LITTLE (V)
MP Ext/Flex	R					
	L					
PIP Ext/Flex	R					
	L					
DIP Ext/Flex	R					
	L					
TAM	R					
	L					
DPC	R					
	L					
Palmar Abduction			L		R	
Radial Abduction			L		R	
Opposition			L		R	

HAND		PROM THUMB (I)	PROM INDEX (II)	PROM MIDDLE (III)	PROM RING (IV)	PROM LITTLE (V)
MP Ext/Flex	R					
	L					
PIP Ext/Flex	R					
	L					
DIP Ext/Flex	R					
	L					
TAM	R					
	L					
DPC	R					
	L					
Palmar Abduction			L		R	
Radial Abduction			L		R	
Opposition			L		R	

Manual muscle testing (out of 5):

		LEFT	RIGHT
Shoulder	Flexion		
	Extension		
	Abduction		
	External Rotation		
	Internal Rotation		
Elbow	Flexion		
	Extension		
Forearm	Pronation		
	Supination		
Wrist	Flexion		
	Extension		
	Ulnar Deviation		
	Radial Deviation		
Hand	Digit I Extension		
	Digit I Adduction		
	Digit I Opposition		

Strength in pounds:

Dynamometer: Rung number _____

	GRIP	THREE-POINT PINCH	LATERAL PINCH
Right			
Left			

Special tests:

TEST: R/L	POSITIVE	NEGATIVE
Allen Test		
Ballottement Test		
Finkelstein's Test		
Grind Test		
Froment Test		
Phalen's Test		
Piano Key Test		
Linshield Test		
Reverse Phalen's Test		
Tinel's Test		

Watson Test		
TFCC Load Test		
Cozen's Test		
Other:		

Scapular mobility:

Postural assessment and structural symmetry:

Functional scale and score:

Occupational performance deficits:

Long-term goals:
  1.
  2.
  3.
  4.

Short-term goals:
  1.
  2.
  3.
  4.
  5.
  6.

Assessment summary and plan of care:

Appendix C: Daily Progress Report

PATIENT NAME	
DATE	

TREATMENT UNIT CODES		TOTAL UNITS
Occupational Therapy Evaluation	97003	
Manual Therapy	97140	
Therapeutic Exercise	97110	
Orthotic Fit/Training	97760	
Activities of Daily Living	97535	
Orthotic Fabrication L Code:		

SUBJECTIVE SUMMARY

OBJECTIVE SUMMARY

OBJECTIVE	TX TIME (MINUTES)
Modalities	
Hot/Cold Pack	
Whirlpool/Fluidotherapy	
Ultrasound	
Paraffin	
Iontophoresis	
TENS/Premod/NMES	
Soft Tissue Techniques	
Myofascial Release	
Scar Management	
Instrument-Assisted Soft Tissue Mobilization	
Edema Mobilization	
Joint Mobilization	
ROM and PRE	
Isometrics	
Eccentrics	
Concentric	
Functional Exercise	
A/AA/PROM	
Functional Tasks	
ADLs	
Ergonomics/Joint Protection	
Fine Motor Coordination	
Orthotic Fitting and Training	
HEP Instruction	
Total Time	

ASSESSMENT

PROGRESS TOWARD GOAL ATTAINMENT

PLAN

Provider Signature: _____ Date: _____

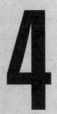

4

Skilled Nursing Facilities

Nicole A. Fidanza, OTD, OTR/L
and Melanie C. Frank-Hirsch, OTR

Skilled Nursing in a Nutshell

Skilled nursing facilities (SNFs) have both short- and long-term residents. Short-term residents are admitted for skilled services, such as rehabilitation, for a brief period and are discharged from the SNF to home typically with a plan to continue their therapy regimen with home care or outpatient services.

Long-term residents often remain for several years because they are unable to recover from their illness, injury, or disease and are unable to function in their home. Under these circumstances, an SNF is a resident's home, and every effort is made to achieve a home-like environment for them. It is for this reason that they are referred to as *residents* and not *patients* in an SNF setting.

Occupational Therapy's Role

Schedule and Productivity

Within SNFs, occupational therapists' daily schedules are determined by the facility's census, the number of residents on caseload, insurance (Medicare, managed care) guidelines, and the facility's productivity standards. Productivity in this setting equates a therapist's time in the building with the number of units billed for that day. Each parent company or SNF sets their own productivity standards, which can be from 80% to 90% for occupational therapists and 90% or more for occupational therapy assistants. The productivity standards for occupational therapists is lower due to the amount of documentation required of them (i.e., evaluations, screens).

Akselrud, R. (Ed.). *Quintessential Occupational Therapy:*
A Guide to Areas of Practice (pp 41-50).
© 2023 Taylor & Francis Group.

Full-time occupational therapists may work 30 to 40 or more hours a week; however, this time may not be evenly distributed across all 5 days. Depending on the variables mentioned earlier, 1 day might have 5 hours of work while another may have 8 or more.

Occupational therapists typically work the day shift from 7:00 a.m. until 3:00 or 4:00 p.m. A typical schedule is Monday through Friday. Many SNFs require rehabilitation staff to work at least one weekend date a month, substituting a day off during the week. SNFs with less per diem coverage may require staff to work Sunday through Thursday or Tuesday through Saturday. Per diem therapists may be used during the week due to short staffing or an influx of new residents needing to be evaluated for therapy services. They may also be called in during the afternoon to assist with new admissions later in the day.

Occupational therapists may spend from 15 to 75 minutes of one-on-one time with residents based on their goals and volition. Individual sessions may focus on activities of daily living (ADLs) (e.g., bathing, dressing, grooming, hygiene, feeding, toileting) and instrumental activities of daily living (IADLs) (e.g., cooking, laundry, medication management), therapeutic exercise and activities (e.g., fine motor or functional activity tolerance retraining, neurological reeducation for postural control and balance), cognitive skills (e.g., memory, attention), or a combination of these.

Reimbursement and Documentation

Due to recent Medicare changes in billing with the patient-driven payment model (Centers for Medicare & Medicaid Services [CMS], 2020), time or minutes with residents is no longer directly tied to reimbursement. Residents can be seen from once a week to daily on the basis of their goals, health insurance coverage, discharge plans, medical stability, and volition. At minimum, CMS requires 5 days per week for short-term residents with 30 minutes per day as one criterion for therapy to be considered a skilled service.

A portion of those minutes can be in a group setting of four residents and cannot exceed 25% of the total therapy minutes. Group topics may include discharge education, balance, exercise, or IADLs such as cooking. Group activities are resident-centered and relevant to each participant's condition and goals.

Occupational therapists are required to record or input their minutes and the skilled services provided daily and distinguish whether the services were provided individually, concurrently (two residents), or in a group (four residents). Other insurance plans often follow the Medicare guidelines for reimbursement; however, it is important to understand the reimbursement criteria in their contracts.

SNFs receive reimbursement for their Medicaid population (typically long-term residents) via a case mix reimbursement system (for those states considered "case mix states"). Payment in this system is measured by the intensity of resources used for resident care. For example, the more minutes of therapy a resident requires, the higher the "weight" of the resource utilization group level, which is used in part for the case mix calculation. Thus, the more resources required to care for a resident, the higher the reimbursement the SNF receives.

Occupational therapists typically oversee a caseload of 10 to 15 residents and share the daily treatment sessions with occupational therapy assistants who help carry out treatment plans and interventions under the guidance of an occupational therapist (National Board for Certification in Occupational Therapy, 2022). It is crucial that occupational therapists and occupational therapy assistants collaborate together for resident care. Depending on the amount of documentation due that day, practitioners may treat up to 10 clients a day with sessions lasting from 15 to 75 minutes. Each day, documentation duties may include daily treatment encounter notes, weekly progress notes (about every 2 weeks or 10 visits), monthly recertifications, discharge notes, new resident evaluations, and screens. Based on a resident's needs and number of goals, these notes may require 5 to 30 minutes each to complete.

Rehabilitation Challenges

In some SNFs, occupational therapists attend weekly rehabilitation team meetings to discuss the residents on the caseload as well as attend individual care planning meetings. They are also expected to provide informal updates to residents' families as needed, either in person or by telephone or video call.

Flexibility is crucial when working in an SNF as the daily schedule is often interrupted and rearranged due to changes in a resident's day, which can include refusing to participate, leaving the facility for a medical appointment, and illness. Therefore, therapists' schedules often are rearranged midday to accommodate for these issues and to enable a resident to still receive occupational therapy services.

Occupational therapists in SNFs face the increasing challenge of providing rehabilitation services to medically complex residents. Those seen for rehabilitative stays may be in the facility for weeks to months following a hospital stay. During this time, a resident is expected to improve and, probably, return to a less restrictive environment.

Whereas many residents aim to return to their prior living arrangement, this is not always the case based on their physical or cognitive abilities at discharge. Common resident diagnoses seen in SNFs include the following:

- *Orthopedic*: Fractures due to trauma such as a fall, joint replacements, osteoporosis or osteoarthritis, degenerative joint disease, and rheumatoid arthritis
- *Neurological*: Cerebrovascular accident (CVA), transient ischemic attack, Parkinson's disease, multiple sclerosis, traumatic brain injury, spinal cord injury, brain tumor, Alzheimer's disease, and dementia
- *Cardiovascular*: Myocardial infarction, bradycardia, atrial fibrillation, pacemaker insertion, congestive heart failure, orthostatic hypotension, and syncope
- *Respiratory*: Pneumonia, influenza, chronic obstructive pulmonary disease, pulmonary embolism, aspiration, lung cancer
- *Hematologic*: Anemia and deep vein thrombosis
- *Genitourinary*: Acute or chronic kidney failure, acute kidney injury, urinary tract infection, urinary incontinence, and prostate cancer
- *Digestive*: Diverticulosis, diverticulitis, gastrointestinal bleeding, and gastric cancer
- *Immune*: Infections (e.g., influenza, urinary tract infection) and sepsis
- *Integumentary*: Pressure ulcers, surgical wounds, and amputations
- COVID-19

Occupational therapists in SNFs must have a strong medical knowledge to understand residents' medical issues. Residents often have medical needs following a hospitalization that require skilled management within the facility (e.g., supplemental oxygen, urinary catheters, ostomy bags, peripherally inserted central catheter lines, wound vacuums). To ensure residents' health, safety, and functional improvement, therapists must know how to work with and around these lines and tubes, as well as understand the medications and treatments used to manage a resident's health. Therapists must be able to take and understand vital signs and identify "red flags" in a resident's presentation.

In addition, occupational therapists must understand each resident's past medical history. Many residents are admitted to an SNF for one issue but have a history of other complex diagnoses, especially dementia, diabetes, chronic obstructive pulmonary disease, congestive heart failure, and CVA. In some cases, a past medical issue that was dormant may exacerbate or be rekindled during a hospital or SNF stay. Furthermore, therapists must understand comorbid conditions as these can affect a resident's participation. For example, a resident with CVA and diabetes may experience low blood sugar during a treatment session. Therefore, it is important to monitor the resident during treatment for signs and symptoms of low blood sugar (e.g., sweating, pale skin, shakiness, fatigue, anxiety, dizziness). Due to the COVID-19 pandemic, therapists are required, at present, to have at least two vaccinations in order to work in an SNF setting. Therapists must become accustomed to wearing personal protective equipment (e.g., N95 face masks, face shields, disposable gowns and gloves) when working with COVID-19–positive residents or persons under monitoring.

Evaluation and Assessments

Residents are expected to be evaluated by various therapies within 36 hours of admission to the SNF (CMS, 2020). Occupational therapy evaluations may be performed alone or in combination with another discipline, usually physical therapy. The more medically complex and functionally dependent the resident, the higher the odds of needing two sets of skilled hands to conduct the evaluation. It is up to the therapy team to determine if occupational and physical therapy evaluations will be completed together or separately.

Rehabilitation departments use a variety of electronic medical record (EMR) applications designed to automate work flow and assist with key documentation components to maximize reimbursement and ensure compliance. All documentation is subject to audit by CMS, the Department of Health and Human Services, and third-party payers. These key components for an initial evaluation (i.e., plan of care) include but are not limited to the following:

- Medical and treatment diagnosis directly related to the planned intervention
- Onset of present illness and dates of recent hospitalization, as applicable
- Prior level of ADLs function
- Prior living environment (e.g., accessibility, family arrangement in the home)
- Reason for rehabilitation referral (e.g., recent hospitalization, decline in function)
- Medical or therapy necessity highlighting why the skills of a therapist are required, including the consequences if therapy is not provided (e.g., dependence)
- Past medical history
- Medications
- Precautions
- Physical and cognitive deficits and strengths
- Results from any standardized tests
- "Section GG" (explained later in this chapter)
- Short-term goals (STGs) and long-term goals (LTGs) with estimated dates of being achieved
- *Current Procedural Terminology* (CPT) codes relative to the skilled services intended to be provided (e.g., evaluation [CPT 97165] for evaluation with low complexity for 30 minutes, self-care training [CPT 97535], therapeutic exercise [CPT 97110], therapeutic activities [CPT 97530], neuromuscular reeducation [CPT 97112], wheelchair management [CPT 97542; American Occupational Therapy Association [AOTA], 2022])
- Prognosis or rehabilitation potential with a brief explanation of why (e.g., if excellent, the resident's prior level of functioning was independent in all ADLs aspects)
- Informed consent indicating that the intervention plan, benefits, and risks were discussed with the resident who has agreed to the treatment
- Frequency and duration of treatment
- Signature, credentials, and date of evaluation or plan of care (therapist signatures *must* match as identified on their state license)
- Signature and date by a physician certifying the need for the services furnished under the treatment plan while under the care of that physician

Occupational therapists must familiarize themselves with the EMR used in their work setting. Per diem therapists may need to know several types of EMRs. The EMR software companies often have tutorials or test areas where therapists can practice. The more therapists familiarize themselves with how to navigate the EMR, the easier the task becomes. New graduates often require 45 to 60 minutes for data entry while experienced therapists require less time depending on an evaluation's complexity and their general familiarity with computer applications.

Moreover, the occupational therapy evaluation consists of an occupational profile created by the AOTA (2020) in order to gather qualitative data on residents to establish baseline functioning for goal setting (https://www.aota.org/~/media/Corporate/Files/Practice/Manage/Documentation/AOTA-Occupational-Profile-Template.pdf). Caregivers may complete this information for residents who cannot participate in the profile interview due to impaired cognition, difficulty with language, or lack of volition. Sample occupational profile interview questions include the following:

- Where do you live? In what type of residence (e.g., house, apartment, condominium)?
- With whom do you live, if anyone?
- How were you performing self-care tasks (e.g., bathing, grooming, toileting, dressing) before your hospitalization/illness/injury?
- What is your home bathroom set-up (e.g., tub or shower, toilet seat height, grab bars)?
- How were you performing home management tasks (e.g., cooking, cleaning, laundry) before your hospitalization/illness/injury?
- Did you manage your own medications before your hospitalization/illness/injury?
- How did you access the community before your hospitalization/illness/injury? Did you drive?
- What did a typical day look like for you?
- What leisure pursuits do you enjoy?
- What type of community support do you have (e.g., family, neighbors)?
- Have you had any falls?

Once the occupational profile is completed, the occupational therapy evaluation focuses on residents' current level of functioning. Every facility or parent company uses their own evaluation tool, which may not include standardized assessments. When standardized assessments are not used, residents' assessments are based on therapists' clinical judgment via observation and includes the following:

- ADLs function (best assessed via a full ADLs session that includes sponge bath or shower, dressing, toileting, grooming)
- Strength (typically upper extremity only, determined via gross or isolated manual muscle testing)
- Range of motion (ROM; [typically upper extremity only] goniometry and contracture assessment)
- Pain (location, intensity)
- Balance (sitting and standing; quiet and dynamic)
- Vision (ocular ROM, visual fields, tracking, saccadic eye movements) and vision perception (neglect or inattention, figure ground, contrast)
- Hearing
- Coordination (fine motor movements, presence of ataxia)
- Sensation (somatosensation, proprioception)
- Vital signs (before, during, and after evaluation)
- Cognition (orientation, attention, sequencing, problem solving)
- Functional activity tolerance (sitting and standing tolerance, need for rest breaks)

Once the initial assessment is completed, occupational therapists generate goals for a resident's rehabilitation stay. LTGs are typically written in 4-week installments and seek to maximize level of independence. LTGs may or may not be written to reflect residents' baseline functioning but rather set the functioning needed for discharge from the SNF. STGs are typically written in 2-week installments and are the "building blocks" to achieving the LTGs. All goals are expected to be written as SMART goals (specific, measurable, attainable, relevant, time bound; Sames, 2015). Goals should include the type and amount of resident cues needed.

When setting goals, occupational therapists must be realistic in recognizing the change from residents' baseline to their current level of function while also considering their medical complexities and prognosis. Therefore, not all residents will return to independence or to their prior residence especially if living alone. Medical histories that include progressive neurological conditions (e.g., dementia, Parkinson's disease) may prevent residents from returning to their baseline function just by the nature of the disease. Therapists must aim for a realistic, attainable goal, which may mean supervision or physical assistance on discharge from the SNF. In general, occupational therapists in an SNF help residents progress from unable to able or from able to more capable using "just-right actions" or skilled interventions to achieve their goals.

For every SNF resident, CMS requires the completion of a comprehensive, interdisciplinary assessment, the Resident Assessment Instrument (RAI; CMS, 2019). This assessment includes the Minimum Data Set (MDS), the Care Area Assessment process, and RAI Utilization Guidelines. The RAI gathers data to help staff see residents holistically and identify their strengths and weaknesses, which must be addressed in person-centered care plans. For long-term residents, the MDS portion of the RAI is completed at admission and then quarterly, annually, and when there is a significant change in the resident.

Each SNF assigns sections of the MDS for the disciplines to complete (e.g., dietary, nursing, social work, rehabilitation, recreation). This assignment varies with facility policy.

Typically, the directors or supervisors from each discipline electronically input the information for their assigned sections into the MDS. This information is then transmitted to the state by the MDS coordinator.

The rehabilitation department typically provides the information for "Section GG: Functional Abilities and Goals," which is currently completed at admission and discharge for all short-term residents on a Medicare Part A stay. This requirement may expand to other payers in the future.

Section GG items for self-care and mobility are often divided between occupational and physical therapists and incorporated into their discipline-specific therapy evaluations or screens. This information is either transmitted electronically from the rehabilitation software into the MDS, or the rehabilitation director transposes information manually onto the MDS. Section GG includes prior level of function, admission performance, and discharge goals and performance. In addition, portions of MDS Section O (therapy minutes and dates of service) and MDS Section I (diagnosis) may be completed by the rehabilitation department as per facility policy.

Interventions

Skills addressed in an occupational therapy session are vast and depend on residents' functional and medical status, goals, insurance coverage, and volition. Sessions can focus on just one area of need or address a combination of skill components. Occupational therapy sessions often focus on the following:

- ADLs (e.g., bathing, dressing, toileting) retraining; introduction of adaptive equipment or energy conservation techniques; tub, toilet, and shower transfer retraining; the creation of restorative nursing programs for long-term residents, and client, family, and staff education
- IADLs (e.g., cooking, laundry, home, and medication management) retraining and introduction of adaptive equipment or energy conservation techniques

- Therapeutic exercise for the upper extremity or core strengthening as applicable to function and aerobic conditioning
- Therapeutic activities (e.g., fine motor or functional activity tolerance retraining)
- Neurological reeducation for postural control and balance and upper extremity retraining following a neurological event
- Cognitive skills retraining for memory, attention, problem solving, and sequencing and introduction of compensatory strategies
- Physical agent modalities (e.g., hot and cold packs, paraffin, diathermy, fluidotherapy, ultrasound, electrical stimulation)
- Wheelchair management for seating and positioning issues, pressure ulcer management, and contracture management

Discharge Planning

Discharge planning begins on the date of admission! Discharge planning is an interdisciplinary approach that involves preparing a short-term client to return to home by identifying needs that need to be met before discharge and arranging supports for after discharge. Before the recommendation for the resident to return home is made, the team must consider the resident's home environment, current level of function (cognitive, physical, etc.) and available supports (family caregivers, community caregivers, etc.). Occupational therapists often perform home safety evaluations prior to discharge and typically recommend durable medical equipment for the home (e.g., 3-in-1 commode, bathtub transfer bench), as well as home modifications (e.g., removing throw rugs, rearranging furniture). Upon discharge, home exercise programs, home therapy referrals, and caregiver instructions may be recommended. Should it be deemed unsafe for a short-term client to return home, other discharge recommendations may be to live with a caregiver in an assisted living facility or SNF where increased or even 24-hour care is provided.

Tips and Advice From the Field

The SNF setting is a great place for new occupational therapy graduates to learn about medical diagnoses and treatments, insurance and reimbursement, and the continuum of rehabilitative care, but it does have challenges. Due to the complexities of both the SNF residents and the reimbursement systems, combined with high productivity standards and frequent scheduling changes, new graduates will require initial support. Many companies offer mentorship programs to new employees, but the degree of mentorship varies by site and company (Fidanza & Bondoc, 2019). Before entering this setting, therapists should understand the following concepts in addition to their entry-level skills:

- Vital signs (taking and understanding)
- ROM and manual muscle test (particularly for the upper extremity)
- The O'Sullivan Functional Balance Scale (O'Sullivan & Schmitz, 2007)
- Global Deterioration Scale (Reisberg et al., 1982; Sames, 2015)
- Basic wheelchair seating and positioning

Additional tips for occupational therapists working in SNFs include the following:

- Have a plan for the day but be prepared for that plan to change multiple times.
- Be prepared for residents or their families to decline the services. Be ready to have difficult conversations about the importance of participating in therapy to remain in the SNF and ultimately be discharged. Knowing resident preferences and interests can help motivate them to participate at a time that works for them.

- Work collaboratively with the nursing staff. Whether during toileting or scheduling a session around a resident's IV infusion, a positive working relationship is key. Collaboration between therapy and nursing is not a given, and sometimes it takes an effort to earn a colleague's trust.
- Be prepared to have difficult conversations with clients and their families during care plan meetings. The rehabilitation team often discusses issues such as lack of progress, concerns about returning home alone, the need for 24-hour care, and results of cognitive testing. Honesty and empathy are necessary.
- Complete as much documentation at the point of service as possible. This not only supports meeting productivity requirements but also captures a session's details in the notes. If it was not documented, it was not done. Be prepared to educate residents about documentation and to explain that the device (e.g., iPad [Apple], laptop) is for documentation only and not for your personal use.
- Listen and observe. Therapists will gain much information from listening, and it can be valuable in helping diffuse situations with residents or family members who may be angry or upset and just want to be heard. In addition, head-to-toe observation of residents is essential to evaluation.
- Practice hand hygiene before and after resident care, which is key to protecting one's own health, as well as reducing the transmission of infections among frail and compromised residents.
- Always introduce yourself and explain how you are going to help a resident achieve their goals because many do not understand the benefits of occupational therapy.
- Make a good first impression. This and a therapist's follow-up will help residents gain confidence in the therapist's ability to help them.

Collaborating With Other Disciplines

SNFs provide for many collaborative opportunities between occupational therapists and colleagues from other disciplines. In fact, interdisciplinary teamwork is crucial to providing quality care to all residents. Staff members partner to advocate for the residents and never lose sight of their needs. Occupational therapists in SNFs work with nurses, nursing assistants, physicians, social workers, physical therapists, speech-language pathologists, nutritionists, respiratory therapists, recreational specialists, and administrators. Each team member brings a unique perspective to the decision-making process and input from all is needed to determine a resident's care plan.

Professional communication among all disciplines is crucial to addressing each resident's physical, cognitive, and psychosocial needs, ultimately allowing for safe discharge from the facility. Of utmost importance for occupational therapists is developing a positive working relationship with the certified nursing assistants (CNAs) who are often at the forefront of client care regarding ADLs and can provide crucial information on a resident's behavior, both progress and regression. They also implement the plans developed by the rehabilitation team, such as a positioning plan or toileting program.

Long-term residents discharged from a rehabilitation program are often referred by the therapists to a rehabilitation nursing program overseen by a registered nurse and carried out by the CNAs on the units. These programs, including ROM, toileting, bed mobility, and eating, are performed 7 days per week and are designed to maintain residents' achievements and prevent further deterioration.

Occupational therapists review or screen long-term residents at least annually. Many SNFs have the rehabilitation department screen residents quarterly to determine any decline in function or potential for improvement. Both of these are also supported by documentation from other disciplines (e.g., nursing), which may result in a referral to rehabilitation services. For practical purposes, many rehabilitation departments follow the same schedule as the MDS quarterly schedule to screen residents.

The state's Department of Health survey team, comprised of trained health care professionals, conducts unannounced onsite inspections of SNFs every 9 to 15 months. This team utilizes established protocols to review documentation, observe resident care, inspect the environment, and interview residents and their families. The purpose of the survey is to determine whether the facility is compliant with state and federal regulations and to ensure resident quality of care and life.

Occupational therapists can play an important role as part of an interdisciplinary team to help residents "attain and maintain [their] highest practicable physical, mental, and psychosocial well-being" (CMS, 1991). By improving or maintaining residents' ability to perform ADLs and their functional mobility, occupational therapists help SNFs who receive Medicare and Medicaid funding to meet the requirements of the Omnibus Budget Reconciliation Act of 1987. For example, the therapists can help prevent pressure injuries by providing wheelchair and bed positioning that includes the use of anti-decubitus cushions, help residents maintain independence in feeding by providing a variety of adaptive devices, assess the residents' ability to navigate the dining table during meals, and provide splints, or caregiver training, to support functional mobility and minimize the risk of contractures.

Suitability for Practice

To thrive in SNFs, occupational therapists must be passionate about the older adult population. Dealing with chronic medical conditions, especially those that are progressive and can elicit resident agitation or aggression, can make working with this population difficult. Therapists must truly admire this population and be committed to maximizing their quality of life in order to prevent therapist burnout.

Another crucial skill is organization. Managing a large caseload, with each client having specific functional and psychosocial needs, can be daunting. Occupational therapists in this setting must keep track of each resident via collaboration with therapy assistants and CNAs. Organization is also required for tracking documentation due dates and setting a daily schedule.

Flexibility is necessary because some therapists split their time between buildings, which may not be planned for a given day. Flexibility also is needed when rearranging the daily schedule due to resident refusals, illness, or appointments out of the building.

In addition, occupational therapists must communicate honestly with their clients, especially when discussing difficult matters, such as discharge plans, failure to make progress, and discharge from the caseload. Communication among members of the interdisciplinary team is critical for successful collaboration toward positive resident outcomes.

Lifelong learning is a must. Occupational therapists working in SNFs need to seek continuing education opportunities on diverse topics, such as understanding certain diagnoses (e.g., neurological, orthopedic, cardiovascular), working with frail older or medically fragile residents, evidence-based approaches for aging, techniques such as manual therapy or neurodevelopmental treatment, vestibular and vision rehabilitation, dementia and cognitive rehabilitation, fall prevention, and understanding lines and tubes. Two recommended textbooks on older adults are *Gerontology for the Health Care Professional, Fourth Edition* (Robnett et al., 2019) and *Functional Performance in Older Adults, Fourth Edition* (Bonder & Dal Bello-Haas, 2018).

A variety of organizations and websites provide current information on SNF trends and regulations and include the following:

- CMS (www.cms.gov)
- Medicare's Nursing Home Comparison (https://www.medicare.gov/nursinghomecompare/search.html)
- McKnight's Long-Term Care News (https://www.mcknights.com/)
- The AOTA, including the Productive Aging Special Interest Section (https://www.aota.org/Practice/Manage/SIS/Productive-Aging.aspx)

- State Occupational Therapy Associations
- National Board for Certification in Occupational Therapy (https://www.nbcot.org/en/Certificants/Certification#Evidence-BasedResources)
- State Health Facilities Associations (e.g., New York State Health Facilities Association, Health Care Association of New York State monthly updates)
- Geriatric Occupational Therapy, Physical Therapy, and Speech-Language Pathology Collaborative Facebook Group, with more than 41,000 members

References

American Occupational Therapy Association. (2020). Occupational therapy practice framework: Domain and process (4th ed.). *American Journal of Occupational Therapy, 74*(Suppl. 2), 7412410010p1-7412410010p87. https://doi.org/10.5014/ajot.2020.74S2001

American Occupational Therapy Association. (2022). *2022 CPT codes for occupational therapy.* American Occupational Therapy Association. https://www.aota.org/advocacy/advocacy-news/2022/frequently-used-2022-cpt-codes-for-occupational-therapy

Centers for Medicare & Medicaid Services. (2019). *Minimum Data Set (MDS) 3.0 Resident Assessment Instrument (RAI) manual.* https://www.cms.gov/Medicare/Quality-Initiatives-Patient-Assessment-Instruments/NursingHomeQualityInits/MDS30RAIManual

Centers for Medicare & Medicaid Services. (2020). *Patient driven payment model.* https://www.cms.gov/Medicare/Medicare-Fee-for-Service-Payment/SNFPPS/PDPM#fact

Fidanza, N., & Bondoc, S. (2019, April). *Expectation versus reality: The lived experience of newly graduated OTs in skilled-nursing facilities* [Presentation]. American Occupational Therapy Association's Annual Conference & Expo, New Orleans, LA.

National Board for Certification in Occupational Therapy. (2022). *Certification—Evidence-based resources.* https://www.nbcot.org/en/Certificants/Certification#Evidence-BasedResources

Omnibus Budget Reconciliation Act of 1987, H.R. 3545, 100th Cong. (1987). https://www.congress.gov/bill/100th-congress/house-bill/3545

O'Sullivan, S. B., & Schmitz T. J. (2007). *Physical rehabilitation: Assessment and treatment* (5th ed., p. 254). F. A. Davis.

Reisberg, B., Ferris, S. H., de Leon, M. J., & Crook, T. (1982). The Global Deterioration Scale for assessment of primary degenerative dementia. *American Journal of Psychiatry, 139*(9), 1136-1139. https://doi.org/10.1176/ajp.139.9.1136

Sames, K. M. (2015). *Documenting occupational therapy practice* (3rd ed.). Pearson.

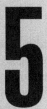

Early Intervention

Rachelle Lydell, MSOT, OTR/L; LoriBeth Kimmel, MS, OTR;
Dale A. Coffin, EdD, OTR/L; Catherine J. Leslie, PhD, OTR/L, MOT, CEIS;
and Heather Page, OTD, OTR/L

Early Intervention in a Nutshell

Early intervention (EI) is the term that describes the services and supports provided to families of infants and young children with or at risk of developmental delays (DDs) and disabilities through the Individuals with Disabilities Education Improvement Act (IDEA) of 2004. EI services can vary from state to state and within different EI centers in the same state.

Typical diagnoses and skills addressed in EI include DDs, attention deficits, sensory-processing difficulties and sensory integration disorders, communication delays, feeding difficulties, Down syndrome, autism spectrum disorder, myotonic muscular dystrophy, microcephaly or anencephaly, congenital heart defect, cortical visual impairment, prematurity, cerebral palsy, torticollis with and without plagiocephaly, brachial plexus injury, and genetic disorders.

Occupational Therapy's Role

Service Locations

EI services are provided in a child's natural environment, where children typically participate in their daily activities. For example, EI services can be provided in the family's home, a day care center, or a community location (e.g., playground, restaurant, physician's office, grocery or retail store, place of worship).

Akselrud, R. (Ed.). *Quintessential Occupational Therapy:*
A Guide to Areas of Practice (pp 51-66).
© 2023 Taylor & Francis Group.

Schedule

Most EI sessions are about 1 hour and incorporate family-centered practice principles, including providing family education and training using a coaching model. This time also can include provider documentation. Some sessions can be for consultation which can last 30 to 90 minutes depending on the family's primary concerns. Every occupational therapist's daily schedule differs depending on caseload and hours worked.

Evaluation and Assessments

When parents, physicians, or care providers are concerned about an infant's or toddler's development, they can contact their state or territory's EI program directly. A physician's note or prescription is not required. The EI program completes an evaluation to determine if a child is eligible for EI services on the basis of the IDEA's evaluation regulations. Publicly funded programs are available in every U.S. state and territory, providing EI services for free or at a reduced cost to those deemed eligible.

Eligibility evaluations for EI services are focused on a child's developmental skills and abilities, as well as on the family's concerns, and are typically 2 to 3 hours. Evaluations are completed by a small team of qualified personnel from the EI program, typically two to four clinicians from varying disciplines (e.g., occupational therapy, physical therapy, speech-language pathology, social work, medicine). Ideally, EI clinicians are assigned to this team on the basis of the child and family's anticipated needs as identified on the initial referral. Typically, EI services are provided to children ages 0 to 3 with DDs or established developmental conditions or diagnoses or who are at risk of DDs within their natural environment and their everyday routines and activities.

Although EI is part of the federal IDEA program, every U.S. state and territory has its own process and criteria for determining eligibility. The Centers for Disease Control and Prevention provides links to every program, as well as information about EI (see https://www.cdc.gov/ncbddd/actearly/parents/states.html).

To determine if a child is eligible for EI supports and services, programs use various methods and procedures to make the decision on the basis of IDEA guidelines, as well as uses mandates from the state where the program is located. For example, in Massachusetts, EI programs presently are required to use the Battelle Developmental Inventory, Second Edition (Newborg, 2005).

EI programs utilize standardized assessment tools to assess children's development, engage in interviews and discussions with families, and complete observations of children in their home or other settings. Examples of standardized measures used for determining eligibility are found in Table 5-1.

Assessments used can be one alone or a combination depending on the needs of the child. Assessments should provide a standard measure of percentiles, standard deviation, age equivalent, or percentage of delay. Tool implementation varies widely by state.

Sample Forms

Required EI forms are specific to every state. Some examples are available through the following publicly available websites:

- Massachusetts: https://www.mass.gov/early-intervention-materials-and-resources
- New York State: https://www.health.ny.gov/community/infants_children/early_intervention/
- New York City: https://www1.nyc.gov/site/doh/providers/resources/early-intervention-provider-policies-procedures-forms.page
- North Carolina: https://beearly.nc.gov/index.php/staff/forms
- South Carolina: https://msp.scdhhs.gov/babynet/site-page/babynet-forms
- Wisconsin: https://www.dhs.wisconsin.gov/birthto3/forms.htm

TABLE 5-1

Sample Early Intervention Occupational Therapy Assessments

ASSESSMENT	PURPOSE
Ages and Stages Questionnaire: Social-Emotional, Second Edition	A parent-completed tool designed to exclusively screen for social and emotional behaviors outside young children's typical "ups and downs." Is highly reliable and easy to screen for important areas of social-emotional competence, behaviors of concern, and any need for further assessment or ongoing monitoring (Squires et al., 2015).
Alberta Infant Motor Scale	Assesses through observation of infants who are delayed or atypical in their motor performance and evaluates motor development over time (Piper & Darrah, 1994).
Assessment of Motor and Process Skills	An observational assessment that measures the performance quality of tasks related to activities of daily living (ADLs) in a natural environment. Designed to examine the interplay among the person, ADLs, and environment (Fisher & Jones, 2012).
Bayley Scales of Infant and Toddler Development	An individually administered instrument designed to assess the developmental functioning of infants, toddlers, and young children ages 1 to 42 months. Assesses cognitive, language, motor, adaptive, and social-emotional development (Bayley, 2005).
Battelle Developmental Inventory, Second Edition	An individually administered, standardized assessment battery designed for children age birth to 7 years, 11 months. Measures key developmental skills in adaptive, personal, social, communication, motor, and cognitive areas (Newborg, 2005).
Bruininks-Oseretsky Test of Motor Proficiency, Second Edition	Delivers the most precise and comprehensive measure of gross and fine motor skills. Easy to administer and contains subtests and challenging game-like tasks for children ages 4 to 21 years (Bruininks & Bruininks, 2005).
Clinical Observations	Measuring, questioning, evaluating, or otherwise observing children to make a clinical judgment.
Developmental Assessment of Young Children	A popular test to identify children (ages birth through 5 years) with possible delays in cognition, communication, social-emotional development, physical development, and adaptive behavior. Five domains reflect areas mandated for assessment and intervention for young children in IDEA and can be assessed independently, so examiners can test only the domains that interest them or test all domains when a measure of general development is desired. Format allows examiners to obtain information about children's abilities through observation, caregiver interview, and direct assessment. May be used in arena assessment so that each discipline can use the tool independently (Voress & Maddox, 2013).

(continued)

Table 5-1 (continued)

Sample Early Intervention Occupational Therapy Assessments

ASSESSMENT	PURPOSE
Early Learning Accomplishment Profile	Provides a systematic method for observing children's (birth to 36 months) skill development and functioning (Glover et al., 1988).
Hawaii Early Learning Profile	A comprehensive, family-centered, curriculum-based assessment for infants and toddlers and their families that provides a comprehensive framework for ongoing assessment, planning, and tracking progress. Domains include cognitive, language, gross motor, fine motor, social-emotional, and self-help. Products are cross-referenced through skill ID numbers for easy linking between assessment and curriculum materials (Parks, 1994).
Infant/Toddler Sensory Profile, Second Edition	Links performance strengths and barriers with children's sensory-processing patterns. Provides a natural way to include families in the information-gathering process (Dunn, 2014).
Miller Assessment of Preschoolers	Designed to evaluate the developmental status of children ages 2 years, 9 months to 5 years, 8 months across a broad range of areas, including behavioral, motor, and cognitive functioning. Test items are categorized into five performance indices. Can be used to provide a developmental overview and clarify strengths and weaknesses for children with severe DDs (Miller, 1988).
Peabody Developmental Motor Scale, Second Edition	An early childhood motor development program that provides both in-depth assessment and training or remediation of gross and fine motor skills. Six subtests measure interrelated motor abilities that develop early in life. Designed to assess the motor skills of children from birth through age 5 years (Folio & Fewell, 2000).
Sensory Processing Measure	Provides a complete picture of a child's sensory-processing difficulties at school and home. Sensory Processing Measure–Preschool extends the measure down to age 2 years, making EI possible (Parham et al., 2007).
Short Child Occupational Profile, Version 2.2	An occupation-focused assessment developed by an international group that determines how a child's volition, habituation, skills, and the environment facilitate or restrict participation. Facilitates a systematic evaluation of most Model of Human Occupation concepts. Ratings are based on each child's "individual developmental trajectory" (i.e., the capacities a child has or the potential to acquire in the future given age, impairment, prior life experiences, and environmental context). Captures each child's strengths as well as challenges (Bowyer et al., 2008).

(continued)

TABLE 5-1 (CONTINUED)	
Sample Early Intervention Occupational Therapy Assessments	
ASSESSMENT	**PURPOSE**
Vineland Adaptive Behavior Scales, Third Edition	A standardized assessment tool that utilizes a semi-structured interview to measure adaptive behavior and support the diagnosis of intellectual DDs, autism spectrum disorder, and delays. May be used to determine eligibility or qualification for special services, plan rehabilitation or intervention programs, and track and report progress (Sparrow et al., 2005).

To find a state's lead agency, visit the Early Childhood Technical Assistance Center (ECTA; https://ectacenter.org/contact/ptccoord.asp).

Progress Summaries/Reviews

After a child has been in the EI program for 6 months, a review is completed to review goals, the Individualized Family Service Plan (IFSP), and any new concerns. Parents can request an assessment in any area of development (e.g., sensory processing).

Children are reassessed every 6 months until their third birthday to determine if they are eligible for continued services. Occupational therapy evaluation, reevaluation, and plan of care documents vary state by state and across programs and is dependent on EI state eligibility criteria.

Sample Goals

When children are referred for EI services, an eligibility evaluation is completed by a team to determine if they qualify for enrollment. The professional makeup of the team often depends on a program's available resources and personnel and varies by state.

Families are assigned a designated service coordinator, who in some cases may be an occupational therapist. Other professionals on the team can include physical therapists, speech–language pathologists, social workers, physician assistants, nutritionists, educational diagnosticians, psychologists, and nurses.

After a child is deemed eligible for EI services, the team, along with the family, meets to develop an IFSP. This process involves talking and collaborating to build understanding of the parents' or caregivers' priorities about the child's development and the family's needs, including the family's relationships, challenges, and strengths and their ability to complete everyday routines, tasks, and activities in the home and community.

The IFSP helps the EI team understand the challenging aspects of participation in family and community activities and directs them toward providing support by recognizing the child and family's strengths and interests. This knowledge is helpful for future therapy sessions and helps the team coordinate other services that the child or family may require.

During the initial IFSP meeting, the family and team creates outcomes (i.e., goals) that will be the focus of EI services. The family can create as many outcomes or goals they consider important for the child and family. The outcomes or goals, which are family directed, routine based, and measurable, can be changed, altered, or ended at any time at the request of the family, and each is reviewed every 6 months.

Goals and outcomes are written in family-centered language, can be either child- or family-focused, and are described in a participation-based or routines- or activity-based context. In some states, the goals and outcomes stated on a child's IFSP are based on their current ability and performance level. For example, in North Carolina, when determining eligibility for EI services, a child's skills will fall into three Global Developmental Outcome Categories:

1. *Positive social-emotional skills*: Ability to get along with others, interacting with adults and other children, playing with others (e.g., turn taking, imaginative play, sharing materials, exploring new play ideas and opportunities), attending to tasks, following rules and carrying out verbal directions, safety and social awareness, coping skills, expressing emotions and feelings, and cooperation and participation in daily routines at home and within community environments.

2. *Acquiring and using knowledge and skills*: Thinking and problem solving through play, understanding early concepts, imitation, object permanence, acquisition of language and communication skills (e.g., requesting help, making wants and needs known), and early literacy and numeracy skills.

3. *Taking appropriate action to meet needs*: Learning to take care of self, using hands and fingers in ADLs, using hands and fingers in play, using daily items appropriately, and moving around independently.

The IFSP outcome page includes the child or family outcome, tasks and progress toward that outcome, strategies to help achieve that outcome, and what needs to be seen to gauge progress toward achieving that outcome.

Writing Functional Outcomes

According to ECTA (Lucas et al., 2014), when writing functional IFSP outcomes, six criteria are considered to determine if an outcome statement is of high quality. The outcome:

1. Is necessary and functional for the child and family's life
2. Reflects real-life contextualized settings
3. Integrates developmental domains and is discipline agnostic
4. Is jargon-free, clear, and simple
5. Emphasizes the positive and not the negative
6. Uses active rather than passive words

On the basis of the child's information from other available sources (e.g., evaluation results, the family's IFSP), ECTA also recommends an additional two criteria be considered. The outcome:

1. Is based on the family's priorities and concerns
2. Describes the child's strengths and needs using the information from the initial evaluation and ongoing assessments (Lucas et al., 2014)

Several sample ECTA-based goals that meet all the above criteria are as follows:

- "Marcus will play in the backyard, getting around on his own using his walker."
- "Leroy will play together with his brother while his mom is making meals and express himself using gestures and words."
- "Kimmie will play with her toys so Grandma can cook breakfast and get the older kids off to school" (Lucas et al., 2014, p. 13).

Child Outcomes

Children's IFSP outcomes should be written using the ECTA criteria including using positive language and reflecting the child's expected improvement in learning through functional participation in everyday activities. These include the family's stated priorities and the child's interests and are stated so that the outcome can take place in multiple settings to increase the child's success with participation. For examples of child outcomes, see Table 5-2.

TABLE 5-2

Examples of Child Individualized Family Service Plan Outcomes

SAMPLE OUTCOME	SAMPLE STRATEGIES AND INTERVENTION FOCUS	SAMPLE MILESTONES INDICATING PROGRESS TOWARD OUTCOME ACHIEVEMENT
Charlie will safely transition from formula to solid foods in preparation for G-tube removal.	Addressing the child's and family's relationship with feeding routines and reinforcing the positive "social" aspect of eating; modeling healthy eating habits and a safe outlook toward trying new foods; addressing environmental context of feeding; addressing posture and positioning for good alignment of her head, neck, and trunk; addressing risk of aspiration; educating family about feeding routines (e.g., feeding when hungriest and most motivated, offering solid foods first).	Charlie tolerates textured foods in her mouth; she safely swallows solid foods; she eats a variety of foods and textured foods.
Bobby will sit independently on his play mat and be able to reach for a toy to his front, left side, and right side during play time while at home with his family.	Core strength, dynamic and static sitting balance, gross and fine motor reaching and grasping patterns, bilateral upper body strength, following verbal directions, play interaction and exploration, cause and effect.	Bobby sits independently; he holds a toy with both hands while sitting; he can reach for a toy while sitting with good balance.
Jack will occupy himself in play and play exploration by imitating actions and interacting with simple and cause-and-effect toys.	Play participation, interaction, and exploration; sequencing; gross and fine motor reaching and grasping; transitional and premobility skills; attention to task; hand-eye coordination.	Jack shows interest in a toy; he engages in play with a toy for more than 5 minutes; he imitates finger plays and simple gestures.
Suzy will explore her environment to interact and play with her toys by transitioning in and out of sitting, crawling, pulling up to stand, and progressing to independent walking.	Gross and fine motor reaching and grasping, transitional and premobility skills.	Suzy independently transitions from sitting to standing; she independently transitions from sitting to quadruped; she can crawl to retrieve a toy or desired object.

Family Outcomes

Family IFSP outcomes can be participation- or resource-based. These reflect building caregiver competence and family priorities, helping families access and use community resources and supports, and are engaging and of interest to the family. For examples of family outcomes, see Table 5-3.

Documentation

Documentation includes daily session notes describing day-to-day progress of the child and observations, occupational therapy consultations as needed, and strategies provided for caregiver carry over. All documentation is written in a family-friendly manner and is meant to carry over recommended strategies discussed in the treatment session. Documentation requirements vary from state to state.

Letter of Medical Necessity

A letter of medical necessity is used for medical insurance companies to justify the need for medical equipment. Occupational therapists produce a letter stating the needs of the child and why they need the recommended equipment, working closely with the medical equipment company to create this letter on the basis of the availability of equipment that best fits the child.

Interventions

Occupational therapy interventions are occupation-based treatment plans that promote change and/or growth in an individual. Interventions consist of a plan, implementation, and review of plan and progress toward desired outcomes. Intervention planning involves collaboration between the therapist and client to guide actions that will be taken toward a desired goal. Intervention implementation describes the actions taken to improve client performance and intervention review examines the intervention plan and client progress. Interventions facilitate opportunities that enable clients to participate in meaningful activities and engage in occupations that resemble real-life situations.

Discharge Planning

Discharge documents include a discharge form and progress note, in which occupational therapists document the reason for discharge. Discharge notes vary by state and program. Transitional planning begins when the child turns 30 months old or when the clinician finds out that the child will be leaving the program. The clinician will also refer them to local preschool programming and provide information regarding private services and community resources as applicable. The reasons for discharge from an EI program could be the following:
- The child is no longer eligible for EI services due to their scores on the most recent eligibility evaluation.
- The child recently moved out of the catchment area.
- The family is requesting to end services.
- The child has aged out of the program.

The therapist also writes a letter to notify the pediatrician of a child's discharge from EI services.

TABLE 5-3

Examples of Family Individualized Family Service Plan Outcomes

SAMPLE OUTCOME	SAMPLE STRATEGIES AND INTERVENTION FOCUS	SAMPLE MILESTONES INDICATING PROGRESS TOWARD OUTCOME ACHIEVEMENT
Participation-Based		
Frank and Tamara would like to be able to take Dawn to her grandmother's house with her siblings.	Managing transitions and challenging behaviors, using public transportation, and making Dawn more comfortable and safer in the car.	Frank and Tamara verbally state strategies to manage transitions and help Dawn self-regulate; they show ability to utilize sensory strategies and tools as needed.
Vivien's family will establish a consistent bedtime routine to help her sleep more throughout the night.	Working with the family to establish a bedtime routine, considering possible environmental modifications, educating about therapy tools (e.g., white noise machine, sensory strategies).	Vivien cooperatively participates in her bedtime routine; she sleeps within a reasonable time after the lights are turned off; she falls asleep independently; she sleeps through the night.
Resource-Based		
Jeri will find child care for her son within 25 miles of her new job.	Problem-solving skills, coping strategies, establishing routines, recognizing available personal and financial resources.	Jeri uses an internet search engine; she compiles a list of child care centers; she makes decisions using logical reasoning.

Tips and Advice From the Field

Schedule and Caseload

Occupational therapists in EI can be full- or part-time and can be salaried employees or independent contractors who work per diem and receive an hourly rate per each client with which they work. A full-time therapist can have four to six 1-hour visits per day or one evaluation and two to four regular 1-hour visits per day. Independent contractors can work for multiple agencies and are responsible for creating their own schedules.

Because travel time usually is not reimbursed for hourly clinicians, it makes sense to cluster visits with families geographically. For full-time employees, the agency assigns the cases, and therapists fit them into their schedule. However, per diem employees may not accept a case on the basis of the family's location or due to lack of schedule availability.

Typically, full-time clinicians work Monday through Friday for 8-hour days and start and end their days at their preference or to accommodate families that request early or later sessions. Most sessions take place at a child's home or day care, so visit times depend on the family or child's availability or the times set by the day care facility related to nap schedules and caregiver scheduling preferences.

Independent contractors also may be employed full-time elsewhere and so may choose to work early in the morning, later in the evenings, or on the weekends. Many families prefer these hours because they do not conflict with parents' work schedules.

Full-time salaried occupational therapists' weekly caseloads are based on the productivity requirements set by the EI center or program. For example, when working 40 hours in a salaried position, a typical productivity demand would be billing for a minimum of 22 hours of face-to-face services with families.

Typical caseloads for per diem occupational therapists are based on how far they want to travel, because they typically are reimbursed only for direct treatment. A weekly schedule for full-time per diem therapists could be 15 to 25 children. Any documentation, such as the required 6-month or annual progress summaries, are completed on their own time. Another downside to working per diem is that if the therapist arrives at the child's home and no one is home or a family cancels at the last minute, no payment is received for this "lost session."

Sample Interview

New graduates or experienced occupational therapists may be asked the following questions in an interview to determine their fit with the EI practice area and employer:

- What skills will you bring to this position?
- What do you think are the main challenges?
- What fieldwork placements have you enjoyed the most, and why?
- How would you handle a parent who constantly asks questions about your treatment sessions?
- What do you think the therapist's role would be in this setting?
- Are you comfortable communicating realistic goals and progress with a child's family?
- Describe a difficult challenge that you helped a child to overcome.
- What would be your ideal treatment session for a child with undiagnosed autism spectrum disorder?
- What type of patients do you most enjoy working with?
- What factors do you consider when selecting therapy activities?
- Describe an experience in which you identified the educational needs of a child and successfully developed a way to treat them.
- How do you organize, plan, and prioritize your work?
- Share an experience in which you used new training skills, ideas, or method to adapt to a new situation or improve an ongoing one.
- How do you think working in EI is different from working as a medical center–based outpatient therapist?

See Table 5-4 for a list of pediatric and family topics to review when preparing to work in EI. A good review of EI service provision is the Division for Early Childhood's Recommended Practices (2014). Because EI is based on provision of indirect services in natural environments using a family-centered practice model (Raver & Childress, 2015), reviewing family-centered care, trauma-informed care, and culturally sensitive practice also can be helpful.

TABLE 5-4

Early Intervention Topics for Review

AREAS TO REVIEW		COMMON EARLY INTERVENTION CONDITIONS AND DISABILITIES	
Motor: Gross, fine, and perceptual	Family-centered care	Prematurity	Down syndrome
Other disciplines' roles	Trauma-informed care	Torticollis	Genetic disorders
Telehealth and virtual sessions	Use of Zoom and other technologies	Substance use disorder	Domestic violence
Coaching interaction style or therapist as primary coach approach	Natural-environment learning practices	Feeding and swallowing issues	Sleep issues
Developmental milestones: Social, cognition, adaptive, communication	Coaching model	Erb's palsy	Behavior management techniques
Administration of typical pediatric assessments	Play skills	Plagiocephaly	Global developmental delay
Therapeutic positioning	Adult learning styles	Neonatal abstinence syndrome	Hearing impairment
Culturally sensitive practice	Caring for a child with a disability	Hypotonia	Vision impairment
Typical vs. atypical reflexes and reflex integration	Interpreting and communicating assessment results	Autism spectrum disorder	Cerebral palsy
Assessing muscle tone, muscle strength and weakness, and range of motion	Community resources for families	Sensory-processing issues	Postpartum depression

Supervision, Mentorship, and Resources

Because of the independent nature of the EI setting, occupational therapists spend much time working on their own. Therefore, it can be helpful for new graduates or EI therapists to shadow an experienced therapist for a few cases, if possible, and to find a local mentor with which to discuss cases.

In EI, occupational and physical therapists are sometimes seen as the "motor therapists" and thus can treat many children with gross motor concerns. Therefore, it is beneficial to have access to pediatric resources specific to gross motor development, diagnoses affecting motor development, and information about assistive technology, seating, and mobility devices for young children to reference during intervention planning and to share with families. Joining the American Occupational

Therapy Association (AOTA) and participating in a Special Interest Section or group related to EI or children, as well as joining the state occupational therapy organization, can provide additional support and information about local and state legislation related to EI.

It is vital to reach out to supervisors and coworkers for support, ideas, or resources. Get to know the EI providers who are not occupational therapists to learn from and collaborate with them.

Recommended books to read about EI and related issues include the following:

- Ernsperger, L., & Stegen-Hanson, T. (2004). *Just take a bite: Easy, effective answers to food aversions and eating challenges.* Future Horizons.
- Fraker, C., Fisherbein, M., Cox, S., & Walbert, L. (2007). *Food chaining: The proven 6-step plan to stop picky eating, solve feeding problems, and expand your child's diet.* De Capo Lifelong Books.
- Long, T., Battaile, B., & Toscano, K (2018). *Handbook of pediatric physical therapy* (4th ed.). Wolters Kluwer.
- Raver, S. A., & Childress, D. C. (2014). *Family-centered early intervention: Supporting infants and toddlers in natural environments.* Brookes.

Recommended online resources include the following:

- ECTA: https://ectacenter.org/
- Division for Early Childhood: https://www.dec-sped.org/
- Zero to Three: https://www.zerotothree.org/
- American Academy of Pediatrics: https://AAP.org
- AOTA: www.aota.org
- Facebook EI and pediatric groups
- Early Intervention Clearinghouse: http://www.dhs.state.il.us/OneNetLibrary/27897/documents/Brochures/4279R0518.pdf
- MamaOT.com
- Complete an Occupational Profile and log into AOTA.org in order to use their most updated template.

Listen and Learn

Occupational therapists should go into each home with an open mind, as each family in EI has their own story. Also, it is okay for therapists to tell a family that they do not know the answer to a question but will bring the needed information to the next visit. Therapists must do their research and be knowledgeable about a child's health history and diagnosis. It is important for families to trust therapists for successful outcomes to occur. Because each family's priorities and concerns can change, therapists must be flexible.

Successes and Failures in Practice

I (C.J.L.) remember the first time I worked with a child with a brachial plexus injury. I had researched the diagnosis with the family, collaborated to plan the intervention, and helped find an expert for a consultation. The family felt confident and knowledgeable enough to go to their daughter's physician appointments and ask questions to obtain the best care and treatment for their daughter. I knew that even after our time together in EI was complete, this family would continue to use the skills they gained to keep their daughter on the right path for a successful medical plan and a bright future. I learned that an occupational therapist's job is not to be the "expert" who brings all the knowledge to a family to fix things, but it is to help a family build their skills so they feel confident and empowered to navigate the medical and educational systems to meet their child's needs.

I (C.J.L.) also can recall a time early in my career when I could have done more to help a family prepare for their discharge from EI. Although the family and I agreed that the child had made great

TABLE 5-5

Common Disciplines in the Early Intervention Setting

DISCIPLINES TYPICALLY WORKING	DISCIPLINES WITH WHICH EARLY INTERVENTION PROVIDERS COLLABORATE IN COMMUNITY AND MEDICAL SETTINGS
Occupational therapists Occupational therapy assistants	Mental health service providers
Physical therapists	Department of Children and Families (also referred to by other names)
Speech-language pathologists	Pediatricians
Social workers	Medical specialists (e.g., those in neurology, gastroenterology, orthopedics)
Nurses	Vision specialists (e.g., ophthalmologists, optometrists)
Developmental specialists	Hearing specialists (e.g., audiologists)
Special instructors or educators	Visiting nurses
Mental health clinicians	Applied behavior analysis providers
DISCIPLINES OCCASIONALLY WORKING	Community-based rehabilitation specialists (special education)
Nutritionists	Feeding and swallowing specialists
Registered dietitians	Members of the foster care system, including foster parents
Music therapists	Assistive technology professionals
Hearing specialists	Adaptive equipment professionals
Vision specialists	Early Head Start teachers
Feeding specialists	Day care providers and nannies
Applied behavior analysis therapists	Orientation and mobility specialists

progress in EI, my role as the "expert" instead of as an equal partner with the child's parents had left the family feeling worried about the future without me as a support in their life. I should have given the family more tools to help build their confidence to be the child's best advocate and be able to seek the best care on their own. That experience changed my outlook on my purpose in EI, which is to give families the skills and tools to prepare them for the future.

Collaboration With Other Disciplines

Occupational therapists working in EI collaborate with family members and an interdisciplinary team. Family members are a valued and vital part of the team and are included in all decision making and development of outcomes, as required by Part C of IDEA. Besides coworkers, EI providers are encouraged to interact and collaborate with medical, educational, and social services providers in the community to ensure that a family's needs are met (Table 5-5).

State regulations regarding billing for visits involving more than one EI provider can differ. In some states, service providers are encouraged to provide cotreatments with two additional EI providers from different disciplines and as specified on a child's IFSP. Therefore, more than one discipline would see the child and family together. In other states, providers can bill only for the time spent completing an evaluation or for an IFSP meeting.

Suitability for Practice

Due to the nature of the EI setting, occupational therapists must be able to work independently and with minimal supervision. Although some EI visits require collaboration with other disciplines and the family, most therapists complete therapy visits independently and with minimal interaction with other team members. Depending on the EI program (whether state funded or community-based), therapists may be required to manage caseload numbers by prioritizing service provision according to medical necessity and therefore must understand state and federal timelines and documentation requirements.

The ability to communicate effectively and adapt to various personalities and learning abilities is key to being successful in this setting. This role requires a high level of critical-thinking skills and knowledge of child development through professional experience, as well as the ability to seek independent learning opportunities to foster professional growth and learning. These skills are typically found in intermediate-level clinicians.

Students or new occupational therapists interested in working in EI can gain experience by completing a Level II fieldwork placement or initial employment in a community program or private employer before choosing an EI specialization. These opportunities will allow therapists to learn the basics of the setting and build confidence in their skills.

Supervision and training for occupational therapists in EI settings can be a challenge. Clinicians may have a supervisor who works in a differing profession, such as social work. Often, no other occupational therapist is readily available to meet with to provide feedback and assistance regarding treatment and interventions.

Some agencies may require supervisors to meet with therapists once every 3 to 6 months. Other agencies schedule supervision for 1 hour once a month, with the ability to request additional time, if needed. Productivity and billing requirements often are the primary barriers to scheduling supervision and training time, and these requirements can vary widely across states and programs. Because sometimes two providers of the same discipline are not allowed to bill for the same visit. if a supervisor is meeting with a clinician to give feedback or advice, only one of them can bill for that time. This issue can create scheduling difficulties and possibly hinder meeting weekly productivity requirements.

EI providers also may be required to complete mandatory courses and trainings as required by state and federal regulatory organizations. For example, the Department of Public Health funds and oversees EI programs in Massachusetts, and during the first few years of full-time employment in EI in the state, Department of Public Health training unrelated to occupational therapy treatment but helpful for navigating how to do paperwork and understanding various rules and regulations must be completed. During the first few years of full-time EI employment, other trainings may not be funded, nor is paid time allocated to attend them. Ultimately, therapists are responsible for attending occupational therapy related training, such as the AOTA Annual Conference & Expo.

Table 5-6 provides some qualities, strengths, and personality types that are important for working in EI, particularly to cope with the aforementioned issues.

TABLE 5-6

Recommended Qualities, Strengths, and Personality Types for Early Intervention Providers

QUALITIES AND STRENGTHS	PERSONALITY TYPES
Interpersonal skills	Compassionate
Strong communication skills	Empathetic to each family's unique situation
Listening skills	Patient
Health literacy, including putting complex terms into simple language and using "teach back"	Motivated
Teaching skills	Flexible and adaptable to a range of situations and settings
Strong problem-solving skills	Confident in occupational therapy knowledge but able to acknowledge what is not known
Good organizational skills, including scheduling, treatment planning, and documentation	Collaborative and can work with many stakeholders and team members
Good time management	Energetic and playful
Good rapport development	Respectful of all cultures, living environments, and personalities
Work independently with minimal traditional supervision	Comfortable seeing parent as the expert and one's self as a facilitator

References

Bayley, N. (2005). *Bayley Scales of Infant and Toddler Development* (3rd ed.). Harcourt Assessment.

Bowyer, P., Kramer, J., Ploszaj, A., Ross, M., Schwartz, O., Kielhofner, G., & Kramer, K. (2008). *The Short Child Occupational Profile (SCOPE) (V.2.2)*. Model of Human Occupation Clearinghouse.

Bruininks, R. H., & Bruininks, B. D. (2005). *Bruininks–Oseretsky Test of Motor Proficiency* (2nd ed.). Pearson.

Division for Early Childhood. (2014). *DEC recommended practices*. https://www.dec-sped.org/dec-recommended-practices

Dunn, W. (2014). *Sensory Profile—2 manual*. Pearson.

Fisher, A. G., & Jones, K. B. (2012). *Assessment of Motor and Process Skills: Volume 1: Development, standardization, and administration manual* (7th ed.). Three Star Press.

Folio, M. R., & Fewell, R. R. (2000). *Peabody Developmental Motor Scales* (2nd ed.). Pro-Ed.

Glover, M. E., Preminger, J. L., & Sanford, A. R. (1988). *Early LAP: The early learning accomplishment profile for developmentally young children birth to 36 months*. Kaplan Press.

Individuals with Disabilities Education Act, 20 U.S.C. §1400. (2004).

Lucas, A., Gillaspy, K., Peters, M. L., & Hurth, J. (2014). *Enhancing recognition of high quality, functional IFSP outcomes*. The Early Childhood Technical Assistance Center. http://www.ectacenter.org/~pdfs/pubs/rating-ifsp.pdf

Miller, L. J. (1998). *Miller Assessment of Preschoolers (MAP)*. Pearson.

Newborg, J. (2005). *Battelle Developmental Inventory* (2nd ed.). Riverside.

Parham, L. D., Ecker, C., Miller-Kuhaneck, H., Henry, D. A., & Glennon, T. J. (2007). *Sensory Processing Measure*. Western Psychological Services.

Parks, S. (1994). *Hawaii Early Learning Profile*. VORT Corporation.

Piper, M. C., & Darrah, J. (1994). *Alberta Infant Motor Scale (AIMS): Motor assessment of the developing infant*. Saunders.

Raver, S. A., & Childress, D. C. (2015). *Family-centered early intervention: Supporting infants and toddlers in natural environments*. Brookes.

Sparrow, S., Cicchetti, D., & Balla, D. (2005). *Vineland Adaptive Behavior Scales* (2nd ed.). Pearson Assessment.

Squires, J., Bricker, D., & Twombly, E. (2015). *Ages and Stages Questionnaires: Social–Emotional* (2nd ed.). Brookes.

Voress, J. K., & Maddox, T. (2013). *Developmental Assessment of Young Children*. Pro-Ed.

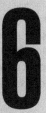

School-Based Practice

Melissa K. Gerber, OTD, OTR/L
and Teresa (Tee) Stock, OTD, MSOT, MBA, OTR/L

School-Based Practice in a Nutshell

About 20% of occupational therapists and 15% of occupational therapy assistants work in school settings (American Occupational Therapy Association [AOTA], 2019b). School-based practice presents challenges and benefits different than those in other settings. School-based therapists, who are integral members of the school team, assist students in becoming independent in activities of daily living (ADLs) or in their "occupations," which includes the student role.

School-based occupational therapy, a related service as defined under the Individuals with Disabilities Education Act (IDEA, 2004), typically uses a model aimed at aiding participation in the educational setting and performance of academic activities. These services also consider student functioning during any part of the school day, including recess, lunch, gym or physical education, and social activities. School-based therapy is not intended to replace outpatient services but to support students while in school.

Occupational Therapy's Role

Students are identified by a teacher, parent, or other team member as needing consideration for testing and special education services. The Individualized Education Program (IEP) team, which includes the student's parents, determines whether a student should be tested, in what areas, and how to proceed. The team may recommend occupational therapy services for students with motor skills difficulties, disorganization, cognitive-processing challenges, visual-perceptual issues, mental health concerns, difficulty staying on task, or unusual sensory responses.

Akselrud, R. (Ed.). *Quintessential Occupational Therapy:*
A Guide to Areas of Practice (pp 67-84).
© 2023 Taylor & Francis Group.

Consultative model services within natural settings, such as the typical classroom, have been found to be most desirable, and many districts are converting to a consultative model for delivering most occupational therapy services (Villeneuve, 2009). IDEA supports services in the least restrictive setting, which often means in the general education setting using a consultative model, to allow students to generalize skills within their typical setting and allow other providers to more easily implement strategies.

School-Based Versus Clinic-Based Therapy

The major difference between school- and clinic-based occupational therapy is the model each uses. School-based occupational therapy uses an educational model that focuses on education and academic performance and is governed by IDEA. Clinic-based occupational therapy follows the medical model and focuses on diagnoses, is prescribed by a physician, and often is directed by insurance coverage. Under the medical model, physicians write a prescription with an *International Classification of Diseases, 10th Edition* (World Health Organization, 1993) diagnosis code and recommend frequency of service. Students who do not qualify for school-based services may qualify for clinic-based services.

Goals Addressed

Students can have IEP goals (Figure 6-1) for nonacademic skills that are affecting them at school or that are important for independence after graduation. For example, a teenager with high-functioning autism spectrum disorder can be on track academically but still have an IEP for social or emotional skills. Some schools may include occupational therapy consultants in 504 or Response to Intervention (RtI) plans.

Caseload, Workload, and Schedule

Caseload refers to the number of students treated while *workload* refers to the activities that support students directly and indirectly. Many occupational therapists are moving to a workload rather than caseload model by reframing their responsibilities in terms of workload. Garfinkel and Seruya (2018) have developed a workload model called the *3:1 Workload Model* that assists with determining the hours needed for direct services, consultation, meetings, and other tasks.

It is not possible to determine a set rule for how many students constitute a school-based therapist's caseload (Massachusetts Association for Occupational Therapy, 2019). Many factors are considered, including the number of students with IEPs and 504 plans and the services listed in these; the complexity of the students' needs; the number of schools and the distance between them; occupational therapy's role during pre-referral; collaboration time with teachers, other providers, families, and the community; documentation requirements; administrative or clerical supports available; and nontherapy responsibilities.

Sessions of 30 to 45 minutes are common, with occasional adjustments to fit the periods scheduled at a particular school. Many therapists cover multiple schools within a district (see Table 6-1 for a sample schedule).

Hours can be part-time or full-time, with full-time varying from 32 to 40 hours per week. Some therapists work from 7:30 a.m. until 4:30 p.m., and others may start later or end earlier.

Ideally all work is done on site at the school, but many new therapists work additional hours from home to ensure they are meeting or exceeding expectations, as well as to research intervention ideas and diagnoses. However, confidential student files cannot be removed from a school building without permission.

Some districts allow short-term occupational therapy as part of RtI, and some do not. Building-level service may be for 12 weeks, with all team members aware of therapy goals due to the short duration of this service. Sessions are typically 30 minutes for push-in or pull-out services.

All goals should have percent mastery, criterion period, how data will be captured, and whose responsibility it is on the team (The International IEP, 2022).

Sensory–Motor Skills
1. Student will maintain attention to classroom activities and not be distracted by normal visual stimuli.
2. Student will maintain attention to classroom activities and not be distracted by normal auditory stimuli.
3. Student will maintain attention to classroom activities and not be distracted by normal tactile stimuli.
4. Student will maintain attention to classroom activities and not be distracted by normal olfactory (odor) stimuli.
5. After provided with a verbal direction, student will follow directions to complete a [number]-step motor task.

Fine Motor and Manipulation Skills
1. Student will complete a variety of fine motor activities for a minimum of [duration] with [number of] verbal or physical prompts across a variety of school settings.
2. Student will grasp, manipulate, and hold specified objects with control and endurance to complete classroom activities in a given time across academic settings.
3. Student will correctly hold a pencil for [duration] while completing a test or classroom assignment across academic content areas.
4. When using scissors, student will use basic cutting skills, holding the scissors in the dominant or preferred hand, to complete classroom activities across a variety of academic settings.
5. Student will pick up [number of] objects using a pincer grasp (index finger and thumb).

Visual–Motor Skills
1. Student will visually track a moving object or an array of objects in a specified direction to localize and focus their attention to tasks across academic settings.
2. Student will complete specified left- or right-sided activities by consistently crossing the midline with no more than [number of] prompts during classroom activities across a variety of academic settings.
3. Student will use near-point copying skills to transcribe letters, words, sentences, or drawings from one source to another piece of paper for [duration] in a variety of academic settings.
4. Student will use far-point copying skills to complete classroom task (e.g., Smartboard, blackboard).
5. Student will trace lines, shapes, letters, and/or symbols within [measurement] to develop accuracy in letter formation and writing.

Bilateral Coordination Skills
1. Student will use two hands simultaneously while engaged in a fine motor tasks for up to [number of] minutes.
2. Student will use dominant hand to write while using nondominant hand to stabilize the paper when writing.

Figure 6-1. Sample student occupational therapy goals.

Intensive-needs classes have programmatic therapy sessions that are a push-in for the whole class (see Table 6-2). Even within a district, schools can have different schedules (e.g., 5- to 7-day rotating schedule). Scheduling challenges include teacher preparation time, building-level math or reading support, and English as a New Language support, when pulling students out of class may not be possible.

TABLE 6-1   Sample School Occupational Therapy Schedule

PARKVILLE

	MONDAY	TUESDAY	WEDNESDAY	THURSDAY	FRIDAY	
9:15 a.m.	3:1 push-in 12:1:1 class	3:1 pull-out Jones	3:1 push-in 12:1:1 class Jones	3:1 pull-out Jones	3:1 push-in 12:1:1 class Jones	
9:45 a.m.	3:1 pull-out Co-teach	3:1 pull-out Jones	3:1 pull-out Co-teach	3:1 pull-out Jones	3:1 pull-out Co-teach	
10:15 a.m.	3:1 pull-out Co-teach	3:1 push-in Co-teach	3:1 pull-out Co-teach	3:1 push-in Co-teach	3:1 pull-out Co-teach	
10:45–11:15 a.m.	Travel to elementary school Day 1	Travel Day 2	Travel Day 3	Travel Day 4	Travel Day 5	Travel Day 6
11:30 a.m.	6:1:2 class Push-in Programmatic—Sensory pathway	8:1:2 class Push-in Programmatic—Movement group	6:1:2 class Push-in Programmatic	8:1:2 class Push-in Programmatic—Sensory pathway	6:1:2 class Push-in Programmatic—Movement group	8:1:2 class Push-in Programmatic—Writing/typing
12:00 p.m.	Lunch	Lunch	Lunch	Lunch	Lunch	Lunch
1:00 p.m.	K students 3:1 Pull-out	1st grade 3:1 pull-out	K students 3:1 Pull-out	1st Grade 3:1 push-in	K students 3:1 Pull-out	Team meetings

(continued)

TABLE 6-1 (CONTINUED)

Sample School Occupational Therapy Schedule

	MONDAY	TUESDAY	WEDNESDAY	THURSDAY	FRIDAY	
1:30 p.m.	Prep	2nd grade 3:1 pull-out	2nd grade 3:1 pull-out	Prep	1st grade 3:1 pull-out	Building consults weekly/monthly
2:00 p.m.	3rd/4th grade 5:1 pull-out	Prep	3rd/4th grade 5:1 pull-out	2nd grade 3:1 pull-out	Prep	
2:30 p.m.*	5th grade 5:1 pull-out	Building level (12 weeks)	Prep	5th grade 5:1 pull-out	Building level (12 weeks)	3rd/4th grade 5:1 pull-out

*The a.m. schedule is 5-day (Monday through Friday), and the p.m. schedule is a 6-day rotating schedule.

TABLE 6-2

Sample School Occupational Therapy Schedule for Karen

MONDAY	TUESDAY	WEDNESDAY	THURSDAY	FRIDAY
8:00-9:00 a.m. middle school (MS) MS1 Day 2 (6-day rotating), Mary 8:15-8:45 a.m. 8:00-9:00 a.m. students MS2 Day 4 Matt 8:00-9:00 a.m. and consults as needed MS2 Day 5 Purple Team consults 8:00-9:00 a.m.				
SMITH Elementary (meeting day)	HENRY Elementary/PR PR meeting day	SMITH (meeting day)	HENRY/PR (meeting day)	SMITH
9:05–9:35 a.m. Sam (K)	Travel to Henry Elementary	9:35–10:05 a.m. Ariel (1)	Travel to Henry Elementary	9:30–10:00 a.m. Ron (3)
9:35–10:05 a.m. Ariel (1)	10:00–11:30 a.m. Push-in K 4 students in sub separate	10:05–10:35 a.m. Bea (1) Chris (1)	10:00–11:30 a.m. Push-in K 4 students in sub separate	10:15–10:45 a.m. Alec (5) 10:45–11:15 a.m. Plan/Prep/Eval
10:15–10:45 a.m. Bill (3)	Travel to MS2 Lunch	10:35–11:05 a.m. Alan (1)	Travel to MS2	11:15–11:45 a.m. Caleb (1)
10:45–1:15 p.m. Plan/Prep/Eval 1:15–1:45 p.m. Lunch	12:20–1:20 p.m. MS2 Purple push-in 6 students in sub separate 6th–8th grade MSMD (flexible for early in the morning 8:00–9:30 a.m.)	11:15–11:45 a.m. Ted (1) Caleb (1) 11:55 a.m.–12:45 p.m. Lunch/Plan/Prep 12:45–1:15 p.m. Ed (2) Mark (2)	12:00–1:30 p.m. MS2 Purple push-in 6 students in sub separate 6th–8th grade MSMD (flexible for early in the morning 8:00–9:30 a.m.)	11:45 a.m.–12:15 p.m. Nora (5) 12:15–12:45 p.m. Lunch
1:45–2:15 p.m. Chris (4) Sara (4)	Travel to PR Elementary	1:15–2:45 p.m. Eval/Plan/Prep/Makeup Elementary schools	1:30–2:00 p.m. Lunch	12:45–2:45 p.m. Eval/Plan/Prep/Makeup All schools
2:15–2:45 p.m. Mark (2) Rob (2)	1:50–2:20 p.m. Lou (2) 2:30–3:00 p.m. Brad (1)	2:45–3:15 p.m. Evan (3)	Eval/Plan/Prep/Makeup All schools	
2:45–3:15 p.m. Evan (3)	John (1)			

IEP meeting with student is made up during evaluation/planning/prep time (pre-arranged with teachers).

MSMD = Middle School Multiple Disabilities Program; PR = example initials of an elementary school.

Some occupational therapists deliver services in smaller inclusion classes, such as 8:1:2 or 6:1:2. In these, students are seen two to three times a week for 30 minutes. Therapists make the goals into class programs and train the classroom staff and teaching assistants to carry out these programs every day to help students generalize the skills.

Therapists can push-in for 30 minutes two to three times a week and do a full class lesson or work with students 1:1, 2:1, or 3:1. The service is written on the IEP as programmatic occupational therapy services with a 6:1 or 8:1 ratio, and the location is in the classroom or therapy room.

Push-in service is dictated by the location on the IEP. If the IEP indicates *push-in to class*, the student receives service in the classroom. If the IEP indicates *school*, services can be done anywhere in the school.

Typical school hours vary among buildings. Schedules also depend on how occupational therapists are hired and paid. Hourly therapists can begin seeing students as soon as they arrive and work until the end of the day. Salaried therapists may receive a prep period and lunch hour each day.

Evaluation and Assessments

Once an evaluation is requested, the special education team notifies the practitioners involved in the process to begin the evaluation. Occupational therapists usually have 30 school days from the signing of a student's consent form for services to complete an evaluation and up to 45 days to meet with parents or guardians to review the results and recommendations as part of a team with the teacher, special educator, and other service providers. Students may be invited by the family or team to take part in the evaluation meeting, especially those nearing the age for transition planning. Every occupational therapy evaluation should include an occupational profile (AOTA, 2020b). Occupational therapists often use observations as part of their functional evaluations. Evaluations should be student and family-centered (see Figure 6-2 for a sample family evaluation) and include student input when possible. Many districts are moving toward evaluations that examine functional skills (e.g., School Function Assessment, Canadian Occupational Performance Measure) as opposed to performance. Many therapists use a combination of evaluations that consider both components (Table 6-3). New practitioners can benefit from having a more experienced therapist review their early evaluations and provide feedback.

Families have input on what areas are being evaluated, often providing this input on an evaluation consent form. Students cannot be evaluated without the written consent of their parents or guardians or themselves if they are of age. Evaluations should be reviewed by parents before their first team meeting.

Interventions

The goal of school-based occupational therapists is to increase the student's participation within the school environment (Frolek Clark et al., 2019). Services should be based upon evidence-based practice and must be provided in accordance with state regulations (Frolek Clark et al., 2019).

Diagnoses and Skills Addressed

Occupational therapists in schools commonly see students with autism spectrum disorder, dyslexia, dysgraphia, learning disabilities, cerebral palsy, Down syndrome, vision impairments, attention-deficit/hyperactivity disorder, nonverbal learning disorder, sensory-processing disorder, executive functioning deficits, mental health disorders, reactive attachment disorder, and other developmental disabilities. In addition, therapists can participate in whole class or whole school initiatives in areas such as obesity, anti-bullying, and other wellness programs. Some therapists are assistive technology specialists in their schools or districts, performing assistive technology evaluations and making equipment recommendations.

Please complete this form to provide us insight into how to best to work with your child.

Name: _____   Age: _____

Past medical or surgical history: _____
_____

1. What are your child's interests or favorite things to do?

2. What are your child's dislikes?

3. Does your child have any sensitivities (e.g., smell, visual, auditory)?

4. How does your child communicate (e.g., express joy, anger)?

5. Social skills—How does your child interact with peers?

6. Self-help skills—How well does your child manage feeding, dressing, and hygiene?

7. Community skills—How well does your child transition within their daily routine and in the community?

8. What are your primary concerns for your child?

9. What are your goals for your child? What do you want them to accomplish?

10. Do you have safety concerns for your child at home or in the community?

Any additional information: _____
_____
_____
_____
_____

Thank you for your time!

Figure 6-2. Parent questionnaire. (Created by Josephine Bardabelias, PT, and Melissa K. Gerber, OTD, OTR/L. Published with permission. Readers can use this questionnaire in occupational therapy practice and education.)

TABLE 6-3

Sample Assessments Used in School-Based Occupational Therapy Practice

ASSESSMENT	PERFORMANCE AREAS	AGES	FORMAT	NOTES
Beery–Buktenica Developmental Test of Visual–Motor Integration (standardized) (Beery et al., 2010)	Measures visual–motor integration in children and adults; sections include visual–motor, visual perception, and motor coordination for writing	2 years and older		Currently on 6th edition
Bruininks–Oseretsky Test of Motor Proficiency (standardized) (Bruininks & Bruininks, 2005)	Areas assessed include fine motor precision, fine motor integration, manual dexterity, bilateral coordination, balance, running speed and agility, upper-limb coordination, and strength	4 to 21.11 years		
Canadian Occupational Performance Measure (nonstandardized) (Law et al., 2014)	ADLs/IADLs	8 years and older	Interview format with student self-rating	Sometimes used for ages 5 and older
Child Occupational Self-Assessment (Keller, 2005)	Functional tasks related to school, home, and the community	6 to 17 years	Self-rating	
Developmental Test of Visual Perception (standardized) (Hammill et al., 2014)	Documents visual perception and visual–motor difficulties	4 to 12.11 years		Has an adolescent version
Evaluation Tool of Children's Handwriting (Amundson, 1995)	Evaluates print and cursive handwriting skills, assesses legibility and speed of handwriting tasks	Grades 1 to 6		15 to 25 minutes, criterion referenced

(continued)

TABLE 6-3 (CONTINUED)

Sample Assessments Used in School-Based Occupational Therapy Practice

ASSESSMENT	PERFORMANCE AREAS	AGES	FORMAT	NOTES
Goal-Oriented Assessment of Lifeskills (Miller et al., 2013).	Assesses functional motor abilities needed for school ADLs. Fine motor includes utensils, locks, coloring, cutting, folding, taping, and organizing and filling a three-ring binder. Gross motor includes putting on and taking off a T-shirt and shorts, bouncing and kicking a ball, carrying a loaded tray, and avoiding obstacles	7 to 17 years		Can be used to determine occupational therapy eligibility
Here's How I Write: A Child's Self-Assessment and Goal Setting Tool: Improving Handwriting Abilities in School-Aged Children (Goldstand et al., 2013)	Student assesses own handwriting and becomes an active participant in setting goals for improvement	Grades 2 to 5	Picture-card interview with 24 cards, sampling various handwriting aspects, with 19 items relating to performance features (e.g., staying on the lines, letter formation and size, letter and word spacing, use of correct case and page margins, ability to accurately copy, and automaticity)	Targets children in RtI or those referred for occupational therapy assessment as a result of handwriting difficulties; criterion referenced with standardized administration

(continued)

TABLE 6-3 (CONTINUED)

Sample Assessments Used in School-Based Occupational Therapy Practice

ASSESSMENT	PERFORMANCE AREAS	AGES	FORMAT	NOTES
McMaster University Handwriting Assessment (standardized) (Pollock et al., 2018)	Assesses various areas of handwriting, near–far point copy, writing from memory, dictation, and composition	Grades K to 6		
Miller Function and Participation Scales (Miller, 2006)	Assesses functional performance related to school participation, and evaluates fine, gross, and visual–motor performance skills	2 to 7.11 years		Can be used to determine eligibility for occupational therapy services
Motor-Free Test of Visual Perception (standardized) (Colarusso & Hammill, 2015)	Assesses visual–perceptual ability without requiring a motor response from the examinee	4 years and older		20 to 25 minutes
Peabody Developmental Motor Scales–Second Edition (standardized) (Folio & Fewell, 2000)	Assesses grasp; reflexes; object manipulation; and visual–motor, locomotor, and stationary gross motor skills	Infant to 5 years	Percentile ranks	Three composite scores: gross motor quotient, fine motor quotient, and total motor quotient
PrintTool by Learning Without Tears (Olsen & Knapton, 2016)	Evaluates and remediates capital letters, lowercase letters, and numbers	Grades K and higher		Free Screener of Handwriting Proficiency

(continued)

TABLE 6-3 (CONTINUED)

Sample Assessments Used in
School-Based Occupational Therapy Practice

ASSESSMENT	PERFORMANCE AREAS	AGES	FORMAT	NOTES
School Function Assessment (nonstandardized) (Coster et al., 1998)	Assesses school function areas: level of participation in six major activity settings; task supports (e.g., assistance, adaptations) provided to student; and activity performance	Grades K to 6	Criterion referenced, judgment based	
Sensory Processing Measure (Parham et al., 2007)	Provides a complete picture of sensory-processing difficulties at school and home	2 to 12 years	Preschool measure for ages 2 to 5	Additional rating sheets for art, music, bus, cafeteria, and gym or physical education
Sensory Profile (Dunn, 2014)	Assesses sensory-processing patterns in everyday situations and profiles the sensory system's effect on functional performance for diagnostic and intervention planning	2 years to adult, depending on version		Various versions available, including parent, teacher, toddler, and adolescent/adult
Test of Visual–Motor Skills, Third Edition (standardized) (Martin, 2006)	Detailed evaluation of visual–motor skills	3 to 90 years		20 to 30 minutes

(continued)

Response to Intervention

Occupational therapists can provide services under tiered models of service delivery, including RtI, which was introduced in IDEA (2004) to identify students who need additional support. Many schools try RtI interventions under general education before referring students for consideration for special education.

RtI often has been described as a pyramid. In the lowest layer, Tier 1, 80% of the RtI interventions take place. This level targets all students with proactive, preventative programs. Tier 2, the second level, is used if the interventions at Tier 1 are not enough and accounts for about 15% of RtI

TABLE 6-3 (CONTINUED)

Sample Assessments Used in School-Based Occupational Therapy Practice

ASSESSMENT	PERFORMANCE AREAS	AGES	FORMAT	NOTES
Visual Skills Appraisal–2 (standardized) (Richards, 2020)	Screens common visual skill difficulties that can affect academic performance and participation, including reading and writing tasks, using 5 items that assess binocular, ocular motility, and visual–motor skills	5 to 12 years		Sections include pursuits (object tracking), scanning (trails), aligning (push-ups), locating/saccadic eye movements (numbers), and eye–hand coordination (design completion)
Wide Range Assessment of Visual Motor Abilities (standardized) (Adams & Sheslow, 1995)	Assesses three areas using three tests: drawing (visual–motor), matching (visual–spatial), and pegboard (fine motor)	3 to 17 years		
Wold Sentence Copying Test (Wold, 1995)	Timed test that evaluates speed and accuracy when copying a sentence from the top of a page to the lines on the rest of the page, which is comparable to copying from a blackboard to a notebook	Grades 1 to 5		Compares speed-to-age norms, examines legibility, forms, and skipping letters or lines

interventions. These interventions are targeted group interventions for at-risk students. Tier 3, at the top, includes the most intrusive interventions and encompasses about 5% of the students referred who are not making adequate progress using Tier 1 or 2 interventions.

Tier 3 programming, which can be done in small groups or individually, is not meant to take the place of special education services (AOTA, 2012a).

504 Plans

Section 504 of the Rehabilitation Act of 1973 protects students with a disability who do not qualify for an IEP (Frolek Clark et al., 2019.) The 504 plan may cover accommodations, modifications, and/or services provided to a student with a disability. Occupational therapists may assist with developing these plans and with helping carry them out.

Discharge Planning and Transitions

IDEA defines *transition services* as a coordinated, results-oriented set of activities that focuses on increasing the academic and functional achievement of students with disabilities to assist with growth from school to post-school expectations, including post-secondary and vocational education, employment, adult services, community participation, and independent living (IDEA, 2004; Stock, 2017). Transition services are based on a student's needs, strengths, interests, and preferences and include related services, such as occupational therapy, instruction, community experiences, and the development of career and post-school adult living objectives.

In 2020 to 2021, the U.S. Office of Special Education Programs reported that more than 7.2 million students had disabilities, about a third of which were ages 14 to 21 years (National Center for Education Statistics, 2021; Orentlicher et al., 2015; Stock, 2017). In 2021, the Bureau of Labor Statistics reported that the unemployment rate for youth with disabilities ages 16 to 24 years was about double that of their peers without disabilities (U.S. Bureau of Labor Statistics, 2021).

Past results from the *Government Census American Community Survey* (U.S. Census Bureau, 2015) have revealed significant disparities in income for those with and without disabilities. Median earnings for people with no disability were more than $31,000 as compared to the $21,000 reported for individuals with disabilities. In 1997, Brandt found that the societal costs of disability in the United States were about $300 billion, including education, medical resources and care, reduced and lost productivity, and premature death (Stock, 2017).

The involvement of skilled occupational therapists who provide evidence-based transition planning services can increase productivity and functioning of students with disabilities, improving their ability to work or attend college and potentially reducing the societal costs of disability (Orentlicher & Michaels, 2000; Orentlicher et al., 2015; Stock, 2017).

An increasing body of literature indicates that occupational therapists have excellent training and experience to assist in transition services (AOTA, 2018; Orentlicher et al., 2015; Stock, 2017). AOTA has published several documents to assist therapists with understanding their role in post-secondary transition planning (see Figure 6-3 for more resources for transitions).

Tips and Advice From the Field

The benefits of being a school-based occupational therapist include being on a school calendar and workday, working in a potentially fun environment, and making a lasting impression on students. Challenges can include paperwork, working out of a small closet or hall space, lack of equipment, scheduling and communication difficulties, and challenges with supervision. School therapists are sometimes viewed as civil service employees and so are not included in the teachers union. Finally, therapists must constantly educate people about the profession's scope of practice to be properly utilized across settings.

Supervision, required training, and the need for prescriptions vary by state. It is the responsibility of therapists to contact their state and national associations to identify requirements for relicensing, recertification, and continuing education. Some states have mandated continuing education requirements per license period. The National Board for Certification in Occupational Therapy requires continuing education to maintain the "R" for registered designation.

Books
- *Best Practices for Occupational Therapy in Schools, Second Edition* (Frolek Clark et al., 2019)
- *Case-Smith's Occupational Therapy for Children and Adolescents, Eighth Edition* (Clifford O'Brien & Kuhaneck, 2019)
- *Transitions Across the Lifespan: An Occupational Therapy Approach* (Orentlicher et al., 2015)

Fact Sheets
- Transitions for Children and Youth: How Occupational Therapy Can Help (AOTA, 2018)
- Addressing Sensory Integration and Sensory Processing Disorders Across the Lifespan: The Role of Occupational Therapy (AOTA, 2014)
- Occupational Therapy's Role in School Settings (AOTA, 2016)
- Occupational Therapy's Role in Schools (AOTA, 2019a)
- Occupational Therapy and Universal Design for Learning (AOTA, 2015a)
- Occupational Therapy's Role With Supporting Community Integration and Participation for Individuals With Intellectual Disabilities (AOTA, 2013)
- Transitions for Children and Youth: How Occupational Therapy Can Help (AOTA, 2018)
- The Role of Occupational Therapy in Facilitating Employment of Individuals With Developmental Disabilities (AOTA, 2015b)

Self-Determination Assessment Tools
- University of Oklahoma Self-Determination Assessment Tools (n.d.)

Tip Sheets
- Living With an Autism Spectrum Disorder (ASD): The High School Years (AOTA, 2012b)
- Living With an Autism Spectrum Disorder (ASD): Succeeding in College (AOTA, 2012c)

Slides
- The Every Student Succeeds Act (National Alliance of Specialized Instructional Support Personnel, n.d.)

Recorded Webinars
- National Technical Assistance Center on Transition (2022): https://transitionta.org/
  - Pre-Employment Transition Services Strategic Planning: A Collaborative Approach Webinar – Part 1
  - Pre-Employment Transition Services Strategic Planning: A Collaborative Approach Webinar – Part 2
- Webinars or online courses from the Virginia Commonwealth University Center on Transition: https://centerontransition.org/training/courses.cfm
  - Job-Site Support: School Staff Role
  - Developing Work-Based Learning Opportunities
  - Building Work-Based Learning Opportunities in the Home, School, and Community
  - Transition Tips: Enhancing Postsecondary Education and Training Skills
  - Employment First for Transitioning Youth

Figure 6-3. Transition resources for school-based occupational therapy practice. *(continued)*

Other Resources
- Accessible Transition Resources for College: http://accessiblecollege.com/blog/
- Casey Life Skills Toolkit: https://caseylifeskills.secure.force.com/
- U.S. Department of Labor—Office of Disability Employment Policy: www.dol.gov/odep
- U.S. Department of Labor—Workforce Innovation and Opportunity Act: www.doleta.gov/wioa
- U.S. Department of Education—Every Student Succeeds Act: https://www.ed.gov/essa
- National Collaboration on Workforce and Disability—Youth: https://youth.gov/federal-agencies/national-collaborative-workforce-disability-youth
- U.S. Department of Education—Office of Special Education and Rehabilitative Services: https://www2.ed.gov/about/offices/list/osers/osep/index.html
- National Secondary Transition Technical Assistance Center: www.nsttac.org
- U.S. Department of Education—Office of Civil Rights—Transition of Students With Disabilities to Postsecondary Education: A Guide for High School Educators: https://www2.ed.gov/about/offices/list/ocr/transitionguide.html
- The 2020 Federal Youth Transition Plan: A Federal Interagency Strategy: https://youth.gov/docs/508_EDITED_RC_FEB26-accessible.pdf
- Transition Coalition: www.transitioncoalition.org

Figure 6-3 (continued). Transition resources for school-based occupational therapy practice.

All practitioners should review the *Occupational Therapy Code of Ethics* (AOTA, 2020a) before starting their job and at least once per year to ensure they are working ethically, including advocating for students for fair and equitable services. For example, for a student whose parents or guardians are unaware or unable to advocate for them, the therapist can speak up if they are not receiving fair or equitable services or can educate the parents or guardians.

Collaboration With Other Disciplines

Occupational therapists working in schools collaborate with other team members, including general education teachers, physical therapists, speech–language pathologists, special educators, vocational teachers, social workers, guidance counselors, vision teachers, English as a New Language teachers, teachers for students with hearing or visual impairments, adapted physical education teachers, team chairs, and principals. Therefore, therapists should have good communication and teamwork skills.

Suitability for Practice

School-based occupational therapists must be flexible, patient, compassionate (i.e., sensitive to a child's needs), organized, and a good multitasker. Without being flexible, the work can be difficult, because schedules change daily. Therapists must be able to adapt what they need and what works for a student every day.

If supervision, mentoring, and training are available, new graduates can be successful in school settings. However, schools are not an ideal setting without feedback and learning from peers or a mentor.

References

Adams, W., & Sheslow, D. (1995). *Wide range assessment of visual motor ability*. Wide Range Incorporated.

American Occupational Therapy Association. (2012a). *AOTA practice advisory on occupational therapy in response to intervention*. https://www.aota.org/~/media/Corporate/Files/Practice/Children/Browse/School/RtI/AOTA%20RtI%20Practice%20Adv%20final%20%20101612.pdf

American Occupational Therapy Association. (2012b). *Living with an autism spectrum disorder (ASD): The high school years* [Tip sheet]. https://www.aota.org/~/media/Corporate/Files/AboutOT/consumers/Youth/Autism/ASD-High-School.ashx

American Occupational Therapy Association. (2012c). *Living with an autism spectrum disorder (ASD): Succeeding in college* [Tip sheet]. https://www.aota.org/~/media/Corporate/Files/AboutOT/consumers/Youth/Autism/ASD-college.pdf

American Occupational Therapy Association. (2013). *Occupational therapy's role with supporting community integration and participation for individuals with intellectual disabilities* [Fact sheet]. https://www.aota.org/~/media/Corporate/Files/AboutOT/Professionals/WhatIsOT/RDP/Facts/Intellectual-Disabilities.pdf

American Occupational Therapy Association. (2014). *Addressing sensory integration and sensory processing disorders across the lifespan: The role of occupational therapy* [Fact sheet]. https://www.aota.org/~/media/Corporate/Files/AboutOT/Professionals/WhatIsOT/CY/Fact-Sheets/FactSheet_SensoryIntegration.pdf

American Occupational Therapy Association. (2015a). *Occupational therapy and universal design for learning* [Fact sheet]. https://www.aota.org/~/media/Corporate/Files/AboutOT/Professionals/WhatIsOT/CY/Fact-Sheets/UDL%20fact%20sheet.pdf

American Occupational Therapy Association. (2015b). *The role of occupational therapy in facilitating employment of individuals with developmental disabilities* [Fact sheet]. https://www.aota.org/~/media/Corporate/Files/AboutOT/Professionals/WhatIsOT/WI/Facts/Workers%20with%20DD%20fact%20sheet.pdf

American Occupational Therapy Association. (2016). *Occupational therapy's role in school settings* [Fact sheet]. https://www.aota.org/~/media/Corporate/Files/AboutOT/Professionals/WhatIsOT/CY/Fact-Sheets/School%20Settings%20fact%20sheet.pdf

American Occupational Therapy Association. (2018). *Transitions for children and youth: How occupational therapy can help* [Fact sheet]. https://www.aota.org/-/media/corporate/files/aboutot/professionals/whatisot/cy/fact-sheets/transitions.pdf

American Occupational Therapy Association. (2019a). *Occupational therapy's role in schools* [Fact sheet]. https://www.aota.org/~/media/Corporate/Files/Advocacy/Federal/Fact-Sheets/OTs-Role-in-Schools-Fact-Sheet.pdf

American Occupational Therapy Association. (2019b). *AOTA 2019 workforce and salary survey*. https://library.aota.org/AOTA-Workforce-Salary-Survey-2019/1

American Occupational Therapy Association. (2020a). AOTA 2020 occupational therapy code of ethics. *American Journal of Occupational Therapy, 74*(Suppl. 3), 7413410005p1-7413410005p13. https://doi.org/10.5014/ajot.2020.74S3006

American Occupational Therapy Association. (2020b). *Occupational profile template*. https://www.aota.org/~/media/Corporate/Files/Practice/Manage/Documentation/AOTA-Occupational-Profile-Template.pdf

Amundson, S. J. (1995). *Evaluation tool of children's handwriting*. Therapro.

Beery, K. E., Buktenica, N. A., & Beery, N. A. (2010). *The Beery–Buktenica Developmental Test of Visual–Motor Integration* (6th ed.). Pearson.

Bruininks, R. H., & Bruininks, B. D. (2005). *Bruininks-Oseretsky test of motor proficiency* (2nd ed.). AGS Publishing.

Clifford O'Brien, J., & Kuhaneck, H. (2019). *Case-Smith's occupational therapy for children and adolescents* (8th ed.). Mosby.

Colarusso, R., & Hammill, D. D. (2015). *Motor-free visual perception test* (4th ed.). Academic Therapy Publications.

Coster, W., Deeney, T., Haltiwanger, J., & Haley, S. (1998). *School function assessment*. Pearson.

Dunn, W. (2014). *Sensory Profile 2*. Pearson.

Folio, M. R., & Fewell R. R. (2000). *Peabody Developmental Motor Scales* (2nd ed.). Pro-Ed.

Frolek Clark, G., Fioux, J. E., & Chandler, B. E. (2019). *Best practices for occupational therapy in schools*. AOTA Press.

Garfinkel, M., & Seruya, F. M. (2018). Therapists' perceptions of the 3:1 Service Delivery Model: A workload approach to school-based practice. *Journal of Occupational Therapy, Schools, & Early Intervention, 11*(3), 273–290. https://doi.org/10.1080/19411243.2018.1455551

Goldstand, S., Gavir, D., Cermak, S., & Bissell, J. (2013). *Here's how I write: A child's self-assessment of handwriting and goal setting tool: Improving handwriting abilities in school-aged children*. Therapro.

Hammill, D., Pearson, N., & Voress, J. K. (2014). *Developmental Test of Visual Perception* (3rd ed.). Western Psychological Services.

Individuals with Disabilities Education Act, 20 U.S.C. § 1400 (2004).

Keller, J. (2005). *A user's guide to child occupational self assessment (COSA) (Version 2.1)*. University of Illinois at Chicago.

Law, M., Baptiste, S., Carswell, A., McColl, M. A., Polatajko, H. J., & Pollock, N. (2014). *Canadian Occupational Performance Measure* (5th ed.). COMP Incorporated.

Martin, N. A. (2006). Test of Visual–Motor Skills (3rd ed.). Western Psychological Services.

Massachusetts Association of Occupational Therapy. (2019). *Guidelines for the provision of occupational therapy services in Massachusetts public schools.* http://maot.org/resources/Documents/56519%20MAOT%20Guidelines2.pdf

Miller, L. J. (2006). *Miller function and participation scale.* Pearson.

Miller, L. J., Oakland, T., & Herzberg, D. S. (2013). *Goal-Oriented Assessment of Lifeskills.* Western Psychological Services.

National Alliance of Specialized Instructional Support Personnel. (n.d.). *Specialized instructional support personnel: The every student succeeds act* [PowerPoint]. https://www.aota.org/~/media/Corporate/Files/Practice/Children/Specialized-Instructional-Support-Personnel-ESSA.pdf

National Center for Educational Statistics. (2021). *Students with disabilities.* https://nces.ed.gov/programs/coe/indicator/cgg

National Technical Assistance Center on Transition. (2022). *National Technical Assistance Center on Transition webinars.* Retrieved from: https://transitionta.org/

Olsen, J. Z., & Knapton, E. F. (2016). *Handwriting without tears: The print tool* (5th ed.). Therapro.

Orentlicher, M. L., & Michaels, C. A. (2000). Some thoughts on the role of occupational therapy in the transition from school to adult life: Part II. *School System Special Interest Section Quarterly, 7*(3), 1–3.

Orentlicher, M. L., Schefkind, S., & Gibson, R. (2015). *Transitions across the lifespan: An occupational therapy approach.* AOTA Press.

Parham, L. D., Ecker, C., Miller-Kuhaneck, H., Henry, D. A., & Glennon, T. J. (2007). *Sensory processing measure.* Western Psychological Services.

Pollock, N., Lockhart, J., Boehm, K., Harrower, A., Hodgins, Z., Leger, M., Blowes, B., Semple, K., Webster, M., Farhat, L., Jacobson, J., Bradley, J., & Brunetti, S. (2018). *McMaster Handwriting Assessment Protocol* (3rd ed.). CanChild.

Richards, R. (2020). *Visual skills appraisal–2.* Academic Therapy Publications.

Stock, T. (2017). *Increasing stakeholder knowledge of postsecondary transition planning* [Capstone project]. Quinnipiac University.

The International IEP. (2022). *Determining IEP goal mastery.* https://www.theintentionaliep.com/determining-iep-goal-mastery-criteria/

University of Oklahoma. (n.d.). *Self-determination assessment tools.* http://www.ou.edu/education/centers-and-partnerships/zarrow/self-determination-assessment-tools

U.S. Bureau of Labor Statistics. (2021). *Disability employment statistics: 2021 youth unemployment rate.* https://www.dol.gov/agencies/odep/research-evaluation/statistics

U.S. Census Bureau. (2015). *Government census American community survey.* https://factfinder.census.gov/faces/tableservices/jsf/pages/productview.xhtml?pid=ACS_15_1YR_S1811&prodType=table

Virginia Commonwealth University Center on Transition Innovations. (2022). *Online courses.* Virginia Commonwealth University. https://centerontransition.org/training/courses.cfm

Villeneuve, M. (2009). A critical examination of school-based occupational therapy collaborative consultation. *Canadian Journal of Occupational Therapy, 76*(1), 206–218. https://doi.org/10.1177/000841740907600805

Wold, R. (1995). *Wold Sentence Copying Test.* https://www.bernell.com/product/WOLDSC/Visual_Non-Visual

World Health Organization. (1993). *The ICD-10 classification of mental and behavioural disorders: Diagnostic criteria for research.* Author.

7

Home Health

*Brett Herman, MS, OTR/L, BCG, LSVT; Kelsey Swope, MOT, OTR/L, BCG;
Jacqueline Ndwaru McGlamery, OTD, OT/L, CCM, ECHM;
Clarice Grote, MS, OTR/L; and Nicola Grun, MOTR/L*

Home Health in a Nutshell

Providing occupational therapy services in the home is a natural environment for clinicians to provide care because of the direct interaction with patients, their environment, and their occupations. Occupational therapy clinicians have a direct impact on patients' daily lives through functional and cognitive interventions, patient education and caregiver training, and home modifications. Clinicians working in the home are most often reimbursed through private pay, Medicaid, hospice and palliative care, Medicare Parts A and B, and private insurance. Providing care in the home can be challenging due to not having the immediate in-person support of a collaborative team, but having the opportunity to make an immediate impact on a patient's quality of life can be rewarding.

Occupational Therapy's Role

Occupational therapists can work in a variety of dwellings, including assisted-living facilities, free-standing homes, apartment complexes, affordable housing, gated communities, and mobile homes. Each setting provides a variety of opportunities and challenges. Home health clinicians must be flexible, as the work includes scheduling patients, creating plans of care, attending team meetings, coordinating interdisciplinary care, and traveling.

Akselrud, R. (Ed.). *Quintessential Occupational Therapy:*
A Guide to Areas of Practice (pp 85-93).
© 2023 Taylor & Francis Group.

Productivity and Scheduling

Productivity requirements vary by employer and setting. For occupational therapy clinicians working in a more rural area, seeing two to four people a day may be a full day's work. Those working in a city center may see five to seven patients a day. Productivity in Medicare Part A Home Health is often based on visits performed vs. time spent with patients, whereas in Medicare Part B Outpatient Therapy, it is often based on time spent with patients vs. visits performed.

Factors to consider when planning a workday to meet productivity expectations include geographic location and time of the visits scheduled, as well as driving and documentation time. With changes in reimbursement, productivity measured by visit may become less popular as employers and agencies explore alternative means of providing care, including case management, remote patient monitoring, and telehealth.

Home-based occupational therapy clinicians work flexible hours, often setting their own schedules. Because each patient is different, considering their times of high or low energy and demands of existing caregivers should be accounted for to promote maximum performance in therapy. Although some patients may need to be "homebound," they are permitted to leave home for medical treatment or occasional short trips, such as visiting a store or hair salon, walking around the block, or attending a family event (Centers for Medicare & Medicaid Services [CMS], 2022a). Therapy practitioners should identify any scheduling barriers to prevent conflicts or double booking.

Travel

In home health, occupational therapy clinicians must consider their commuting time and personal breaks when planning their schedules. It can be challenging to locate a bathroom, food, service stations, or an internet connection. Seeing patients in one geographic area allows clinicians to be the most efficient.

In their vehicles, clinicians often keep a hands-free phone holder, phone and tablet chargers, adaptive and vitals equipment, food and drinks, jumper cables, spare tires, and blankets. Vehicle health should be considered before entering this setting, as transportation should be reliable. Having a backup plan for when a cell phone dies or loses reception when navigating is important. Confirming addresses and cross-streets before traveling to patients' homes can help reduce any difficulties.

Safety and Infection Control

Safety is a key concern for occupational therapy clinicians, who are often alone when entering a patient's home, or when on the road. Clinicians must consider safety practices for illicit materials, weapons, aggressive physical or verbal behavior, and animals. In addition, clinicians must identify and report neglect or abuse on the basis of guidelines outlined by the agency and state.

Clinicians should engage in good hand hygiene before, during, and after visits, and all equipment should be sanitized after every use. Disinfectant and insect repellent may be beneficial but should not be used around patients as their use may be perceived as offensive, potentially jeopardizing the therapeutic relationship.

Reimbursement

Being knowledgeable about reimbursement and quality metrics ensures that occupational therapy clinicians are providing value to their employers and patients. Clinicians who are not informed about reimbursement have an increased risk of denied claims, which is problematic to employers and patients, both of whom may be responsible for the bill. Occupational therapy documentation must clearly indicate medical necessity and provision of a skilled service for each visit (CMS, 2021a).

TABLE 7-1

Sample Equipment Used in Home Health Occupational Therapy

EQUIPMENT USE	EQUIPMENT TYPE	
Assessment	• Pulse oximeter • Manual blood pressure cuff (regular, extra large) • Stethoscope	• Automatic blood pressure device • Thermometer • Goniometer • Dynamometer
Safety	• Gloves • Alcohol swabs • Hand sanitizer • Nasal mask • Pad to place bag on • Insect repellent	• CPR equipment • Gait belt • General disinfectant spray • Plastic stool • Disinfectant wipes (for *Clostridioides difficile*, methicillin-resistant *Staphylococcus aureus*, general)
Adaptive	• Reacher • Sock aid • Dressing stick • Foam tube grip	• Long-handled shoe horn • Button hook • Toileting aid • Leg lifter
Fine motor	• Playing cards • Puzzles	• Coloring pages • Therapy putty
Gross motor	• Therapy bands • Balloons • Dumb bells or soup cans	• Soft balls in various sizes • Pillow for balance

Understanding Medicare guidelines outside of employer-provided education is important for all occupational therapy clinicians, especially those operating under their own National Provider Identifier. Under Medicare Part A, home health agencies are reimbursed through a case-mix adjustment payment based on information gathered during the Outcome Assessment and Information Set (OASIS; CMS, 2022b); therefore, therapy visits are not individually reimbursed. This payment change took effect January 1, 2020, as part of the Patient-Driven Groupings Model (PDGM; CMS, 2018). Under Medicare Part B, visits are reimbursed in units with *Current Procedural Terminology* codes, and must incorporate billing modifiers as needed (CMS, 2021a).

Recommended Equipment

Home health occupational therapy clinicians predominantly use objects in the home during visits to allow patients to engage with their environment in a natural, patient-centered way. Obtaining a sturdy bag is the first vital piece of equipment needed in home health. Table 7-1 lists other potentially useful equipment. If creating splints or treating wounds or lymphedema, clinicians will require different equipment and supplies.

Evaluation and Assessments

Occupational therapy home health visits predominantly consist of initial evaluations, 30-day functional reassessments and progress notes, OASIS completion, supervision of an occupational therapy assistant or home health aide, or occupational therapy discharge evaluations. Occupational therapy assistants are often utilized in home health to carry out the day-to-day interventions under the supervision of a licensed occupational therapist. Each visit should be seen as an opportunity to assess if the next visit is necessary or if a patient is ready for discharge. Medical necessity and evidence of skill must be specified in every document.

During any visit, occupational therapy practitioners are required to communicate with patients' physicians regarding incidents, such as falls, rehospitalizations, changes in condition or plan of care, or death (Federal Register, 2017). Home health agencies often adopt similar guidelines for non-Medicare patients as well.

Clinicians' evaluations begin the moment they arrive at the home. Practitioners should note the home's condition, the walkways and entrances, odors, and animals. Once patients open their door, clinicians can see how well they move, what equipment they are using, any environmental hazards, the conditions inside the home, and general behavior.

The occupational therapy evaluation process is a combination of clinical judgment, administering objective measures that assess patients' interactions with their environment and its impact on how they perform meaningful and purposeful activities, and creating an appropriate, personalized plan of care with goals considering patient deficits and concerns. Although much can be gathered from a subjective interview, direct observation of patient behaviors and activities can ensure an accurate functional assessment (CMS, 2022b) and can allow clinicians to demonstrate progress, show occupational therapy's unique value, and positively affect quality outcomes.

Occupational therapy patient evaluations should include an occupational profile (American Occupational Therapy Association [AOTA], 2020), including caregiver support and living environment, review of the patient's prior level of function and reason for referral to occupational therapy, and standardized and objective measurements of a patient's activities of daily living, instrumental activities of daily living, cognitive function, engagement, falls, and home safety (AOTA, 2020). Evaluations should also document goals, patient diagnosis, and medical necessity (CMS, 2022a). For patients treated under Medicare Part A, scoring of the OASIS functional items, Section M1800, and Section GG should be incorporated into the evaluation (CMS, 2022b).

Personalized patient goals, which are determined from patient-stated focus areas and results from assessments and intake, should be developed in collaboration with patients and be client-driven, occupation-based, and evidence-informed. Goals can include caregiver training. Some examples of typical goals follow:

- Patient will improve bilateral upper extremity strength to 4+/5 to increase strength to independently stand and retrieve items from the kitchen cabinet in 4 weeks.
- Patient will perform upper and lower body dressing with minimum (< 25%) assistance from a caregiver in 4 weeks.
- Patient will demonstrate ability to manage their chronic cardiac condition by accurately measuring blood pressure, taking blood pressure medication, and recording results 90% of the time to reduce risk of rehospitalization.
- Caregiver will demonstrate ability to independently provide verbal cues to patient during morning routine to facilitate patient engagement in self-care in 2 weeks.
- Patient will improve 30-second sit-to-stand results to 13 transfers in 90 days, demonstrating improved bilateral lower extremity strength and cardiovascular endurance to facilitate independence with functional transfers (Rikli & Jones, 1999).
- Patient will demonstrate ability to empty dishwasher with energy conservation techniques and breathing strategies to reduce the risk of chronic obstructive pulmonary disease exacerbation in 30 days.

Although occupational therapy evaluations are primarily focused on determining patients' current level of function, interventions should involve making patients safer in their homes. With changes in reimbursement, occupational therapy practitioners are expected to have better outcomes with fewer visits, so ensuring an optimal return is key. In addition, therapists must consider how comorbidities can affect functional outcomes and adjust the plan of care accordingly. Implementation of diagnosis-specific evidence-based practice is critical.

Occupational therapists should collaborate with the treatment team members when establishing frequency of visits and length of the plan of care to ensure that patients are accessing necessary care at the appropriate time. After completing an evaluation, CMS mandates that a registered nurse or qualified practitioner, such as an occupational therapist, obtain and document orders obtained from physicians following an evaluation and as needed throughout the duration of the plan of care (CMS, 2022b).

Interventions

Standard or daily visits typically consist of interventions that facilitate progress toward patient-stated goals. Each visit should be patient-centered, occupation-based, evidence-based, and driven by the plan of care. The plan of care should identify the type of services to be provided and the frequency of the visits on the plan of care (CMS, 2022a).

Documenting how the visit involved skilled care is critical for justifying the need for occupational therapy services. It is not sufficient to document only objective statements about the visit, how the interventions were both skilled and helped patients progress toward their goals is needed. Examples of documenting skilled intervention include but are not limited to level and type of assistance (verbal vs. physical cues) provided, activity set-up, and any objective information (e.g., exercise repetitions, standing endurance, tasks completed, environmental conditions, patient response to activity, equipment used; AOTA, 2018).

Working in the home allows clinicians to use occupation as a means of intervention. For example, for a patient who wants to pick up their mail or newspaper, the clinician can practice the actual task vs. simulating it. Typical areas addressed can include home modifications, equipment training, caregiver training, chronic disease management, functional cognition, low vision modifications and training, and activities of daily living and instrumental activities of daily living (AOTA, 2020).

Reassessment and Discharge Planning

Reassessments must be completed to justify medical necessity for continued skilled services, to assess changes in performance, and to supervise occupational therapy assistants. Any standardized assessments should be reassessed, and occupational therapists should note the goals that have been met, were discontinued, or are in progress. For patients who have a change in status (e.g., fall, illness) that did not require hospitalization, completing a reassessment or reevaluation may be warranted. A physician or allowed practitioner must sign continuation orders for any changes to the plan of care (42 C.F.R. § 484.60, 2022).

Important aspects to document during a reassessment include the need for skilled occupational therapy intervention, barriers to progress and how to address these, actual progress toward goals, functional outcomes, and patient statements about how they feel occupational therapy has helped them. Medical necessity must be clearly documented to reduce the risk of claim denials (CMS, 2021b).

For patients who have met all their goals, who no longer wish to continue therapy, or who no longer need skilled therapy, occupational therapists will complete a treatment note and discharge summary. In this summary, which is similar to a progress note, therapists must address progress toward all goals and any areas that declined or did not change should be explained. Depending on if the patient is continuing to see other clinicians, a discharge OASIS may need to be completed.

Tips and Advice From the Field

Starting a career in home-based care can be challenging. Clinicians can find themselves in the field without immediate support. Occupational therapy practitioners interested in entering home care will be most successful if intrinsically motivated, have excellent communication and time management skills, and are independent. Because clinicians have great control over their schedules, good time management will allow practitioners to optimally meet patient needs, meet productivity standards, and maintain a good work–life balance. Excellent communication will facilitate trust with patients and other team members.

Mentorship is critical for home-based practitioners because few opportunities exist to directly learn and observe other clinicians as they work. Building a network of support can facilitate success and increase confidence.

Home-based occupational therapy practitioners are typically generalists with a wide knowledge base of various medical conditions. Clinicians also should be aware of medical procedures, post-surgical precautions, vitals ranges, and the types of care provided in other settings. Because it is common for clinicians to have received little information about medical history or documentation for patients, having a background in acute care or other post-acute facilities can be beneficial for understanding precautions and recovery expectations for various procedures and illnesses.

Numerous opportunities exist to address primary and preventative care interventions in the home for many diagnoses. For example, for patients hospitalized for a fall, it is crucial to determine why the fall occurred. Was it oxygen desaturation due to a patient not wearing their portable oxygen? Was their blood sugar out of control after forgetting to take their insulin? Did they take the medication incorrectly? These factors are important to identify and communicate with the team.

Continuing Education and Helpful Resources

AOTA has numerous resources for home care practitioners, including evidence-based fact sheets, practice guidelines, and continuing education on regulations in home health. In addition, AOTA hosts the Home and Community Health Special Interest Section, which is dedicated to educating and providing support to home occupational therapy clinicians. The National Association of Home Care and Hospice also provide support and education. Membership in these associations is required to access all resources, but many are free or open accessible.

The 2016 textbook *Home Health: A Guide for Occupational Therapy Practice* by Karen Vance, BSOT, is a comprehensive guide for new or experienced clinicians. Reviewing CMS documents, such as the OASIS-E Manual or the Medicare Benefit and Claims Manuals, will provide clinicians with an accurate resource that explains scoring methodology and reimbursement guidelines. In addition, numerous Facebook groups, podcasts, and other resources are available to provide support and recommendations. However, as with any resource, it is always recommended clinicians seek information directly from the source, such as CMS, Department of Health and Human Services, or other payers, as there is often a lot of misinformation on what Medicare does or does not cover and regulations impacting occupational therapy practice.

Collaboration With Other Disciplines

Home care team members vary on the basis of payer source and patient diagnosis, acuity, and prior and current levels of function. Team members may include physical therapy clinicians, speech-language pathologists, respiratory therapists, skilled nurses, medical social workers, occupational therapy practitioners, physicians, specialists, and home health aides.

Interprofessional collaboration is imperative when treating patients in any setting to improve clinical outcomes and ensure adequate access to care (Toto, 2006). During these collaborations, occupational therapy clinicians can advocate for the value of occupational therapy services and provide education on how the profession can improve outcomes. Collaborating with other disciplines allows practitioners to coordinate appropriate discharge recommendations, refer to needed community resources, and assist with providing necessary support for current patient needs.

Clinicians update the interprofessional team with patient status changes, progress toward or changes in goals, and discharge plans. Using the occupational therapy practitioner's unique perspective and knowledge base to educate patients and the team about the patient can help patients achieve their best outcomes.

Suitability for Practice

New occupational therapy graduates can be successful in a home-based setting with appropriate mentorship due to their fresh exposure to evidence-based practice, occupation-based interventions, client-centered care, and other useful tools. New graduates often do not feel constrained by limitations that may have been experienced by therapists in other settings. The downside of home health is the clinician is often out in the field alone unlike other settings where there is more opportunity to collaborate with a team or ask someone for help. Although a clinician travels alone, traditional home health often involves a care team and case meetings as the patient is often receiving multiple services at once.

Additionally, the reimbursement structure under Medicare Part A incentivizes increased coordination of care between disciplines to promote high quality outcomes and optimal patient improvements. Another supporting factor for interdisciplinary care is the OASIS and other home health assessments which are intended to be an interdisciplinary assessment that requires increased coordination. The care team is more diverse in traditional home health because CMS covers nursing, social work, case management, home health, and all three therapies (CMS, 2022a). Therefore, the therapy practitioner may have more opportunity to learn from a diverse group of practitioners.

In mobile outpatient or occupational therapy in the home, it is not uncommon for a patient to only be receiving care from one discipline. Many mobile outpatient companies are small businesses and may only involve one or two other employees. If working for a larger mobile outpatient company, there may be better opportunities. Additionally, the reimbursement for mobile outpatient does not cover nursing or social work services so if there are multiple employees, there may only be a couple of therapy disciplines working for the company. Additionally, there are not any required interdisciplinary assessments or regulatory-based incentives for case management, so clinicians working in mobile outpatient settings may not have as many opportunities to interact with or learn from other clinicians.

For occupational therapy assistants seeking to enter this field, working for a traditional home health agency may be the only viable option. This is due to supervision requirements for Medicare beneficiaries. Under Medicare Part A, or traditional home health, occupational therapy assistants must receive general supervision, unless state supervision requirements are more stringent. General supervision requires the supervising occupational therapy be available either in person or through virtual means (CMS, 2022a).

Occupational therapy assistants wanting to work in mobile outpatient private practice billed under Medicare B will have a difficult time finding a full-time job. Medicare Part B requires that occupational therapy assistant services provided through a private practice must have direct supervision, unless state supervision requirements are more stringent. CMS defines direct supervision as meaning the supervising occupational therapist must be in the office suite and available for supervision (CMS, 2022c). So, unless the occupational therapist and occupational therapy assistant went out on a visit together, the occupational therapy assistant would not receive sufficient supervision. Other payers may have less restrictive supervision requirements.

Working in a home health setting can provide a lot of flexibility, but it also requires attention to detail, organization, and independent work. If the practitioner is seeking a setting where there will be consistent in-person support and assistance, home health may not be a good fit.

Medicare Part A Home Health

Home health billed under Medicare Part A is what is most commonly thought of as "traditional" home health. Medicare beneficiaries are eligible for home health services under Medicare Part A if they are homebound and require intermittent skilled nursing and physical, speech, or occupational therapies. Occupational therapy does not establish eligibility for home health under Medicare Part A, so patients must also require another service at the start of the home health episode (Federal Register, 2017).

Medicare defines *homebound* as:

The patient has trouble leaving the home without help such as using a cane, wheelchair, walker, or crutches; special transportation; or help from another person because of an illness or injury, or leaving the home isn't recommended because of their condition and leaving the home requires considerable effort and they have a normal inability to leave the home. (CMS, 2022a)

Beneficiaries are unable to receive both Part A and B services at the same time (Department of Health and Human Services, 2020). Occupational therapy must be considered "reasonable and necessary," and a patient's condition must require either a restorative program that improves function that was affected by the patient's illness or injury or a maintenance program to maintain their current condition or prevent that condition from worsening (CMS, 2022a).

Patient-Driven Groupings Model

As of January 1, 2020, PDGM took effect and eliminated therapy thresholds in favor of a case-mix adjusted payment determined by a patient's primary diagnosis indicating the need for home health, contributing comorbidities, functional limitations, and admission source and timing (CMS, 2018). PDGM is part of the movement toward value-based care and away from fee-for-service–based care.

Occupational therapy practitioners have a unique contribution under PDGM given the increased emphasis on function. The functional impairment section is scored primarily through the M1800s section of OASIS, which includes grooming, current ability to safely dress the upper and lower body, bathing, toilet transferring, ambulation and locomotion, and risk for hospitalization (CMS, 2018). These categories are subject to change, and the changes are published by CMS.

The evaluating clinician establishes the plan of care for their discipline and visit frequency. Medicare does not place a limitation on the number of medically necessary therapy visits that can be provided during a home health episode (CMS, 2021a). When communicating a therapy plan of care, occupational therapists should communicate medical necessity and how occupational therapy services will address patient deficits. Communicating occupational therapy's value is an opportunity to advocate for patient access to necessary medical services.

Outcomes and Assessment Information Set

Under Medicare Part A, clinicians must complete the OASIS during the start of care, at recertification, and at discharge. Occupational therapists, registered nurses, physical therapists, and speech–language pathologists are the only individuals that can initiate OASIS Start of Care (CMS, 2022b). Early involvement of occupational therapy is essential for accuracy of OASIS coding to optimize reimbursement and documented clinical outcomes (Vance, 2019). The most recent *OASIS Guidance Manual* (CMS, 2022b) should be consulted for the most accurate scoring of functional items.

Medicare Part B Outpatient Therapy

It is becoming more common for occupational therapy practitioners to provide services as outpatient therapists but in a home setting. Typically, these services are billed under Medicare Part B. When billing outpatient services, occupational therapy is considered a qualifying service, the OASIS is not required, and a typical occupational therapy evaluation is sufficient. Whereas other disciplines may be seeing a patient as well and interdisciplinary collaboration remains important, the care team is often less expensive than that from an agency providing traditional home health care.

Reimbursement is driven by *Current Procedural Terminology* (or *CPT*) codes, and occupational therapists must consider any modifiers or billing thresholds associated with this type of billing (CMS, 2021b, 2022c). Typically, practitioners will be operating under their own National Provider Identifier and may be subject to quality metrics and requirements of the Medicare Incentive Payment System depending on the size of the practice (CMS, 2021c). More information on these regulations and requirements can be found on Medicare's website (www.CMS.gov) and in its *Claims Processing Manual* (CMS, 2021b).

References

American Occupational Therapy Association. (2018). Guidelines for documentation occupational therapy. *American Journal of Occupational Therapy, 72*(Suppl. 2), 7212410010p1-7212410010p7. https://doi.org/10.5014/ajot.2018.72S203

American Occupational Therapy Association. (2020). Occupational therapy practice framework: Domain and process (4th ed.). *American Journal of Occupational Therapy, 74*(Suppl. 2), 7412410010p1-7412410010p87. https://doi.org/10.5014/ajot.2020.74S2001

Centers for Medicare & Medicaid Services. (2018). *Centers for Medicare & Medicaid Services Patient-Driven Groupings Model* [PDF]. https://www.cms.gov/Medicare/Medicare-Fee-for-Service-Payment/HomeHealthPPS/Downloads/Overview-of-the-Patient-Driven-Groupings-Model.pdf

Centers for Medicare & Medicaid Service. (2021a). *The role of therapy under the Home Health Patient-Driven Groupings Model (PDGM).* https://www.cms.gov/files/document/se20005.pdf

Centers for Medicare & Medicaid Services. (2021b). Part B outpatient rehabilitation and CORF/OPT service. In Centers for Medicare & Medicaid Services, *Medicare claims processing manual.* Author.

Centers for Medicare & Medicaid Services. (2021c). Home health agency billing. In Centers for Medicare & Medicaid Services, *Medicare claims processing manual.* Author.

Centers for Medicare & Medicaid Services. (2022a). Home health services. In Centers for Medicare & Medicaid Services, *Medicare benefit policy manual* (rev. 11447). Author.

Centers for Medicare & Medicaid Services. (2022b). *Outcomes and assessment information set (OASIS-E) manual.* Author.

Centers for Medicare & Medicaid Services. (2022c). Covered Medical and other health services. In Centers for Medicare & Medicaid Services, *Medicare benefit policy manual* (rev. 11447). Author.

Code for Federal Regulations (2022). *§ 484.60 Condition of participation: Care planning, coordination of services, and quality of care.* https://www.ecfr.gov/current/title-42/chapter-IV/subchapter-G/part-484/subpart-B/section-484.60

Department of Health and Human Services. (2020). *Quality performance category: Traditional MIPS requirements.* https://qpp.cms.gov/mips/quality-measures?py=2020

Federal Register. (2017). *Medicare and Medicaid program: Conditions of participation for home health agencies.* https://www.federalregister.gov/d/2017-00283

Rikli, R. E., & Jones, C. J. (1999). Functional fitness normative scores for community residing older adults ages 60–94. *Journal of Aging and Physical Activity, 7*(2), 160–179. https://doi.org/10.1123/japa.7.2.162

Toto, P. E. (2006). Success through teamwork in the home health setting: The role of occupational therapy. *Home Health Care Management and Practice, 19*(1), 31–37. https://doi.org/10.1177/1084822306292230

Vance, K. (Ed.). (2016). *Home health: A guide of occupational therapy practice.* AOTA Press.

Vance, K. (2019). Occupational therapy and data collection in home health. HHQI National Campaign. https://hhqi.wordpress.com/2019/04/19/occupational-therapy-and-data-collection-in-home-health

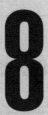

Mental Health

Kristy Gulotta, MS, OTR/L, BCMH, CGCP; Henry Hanif, MA, OTR/L;
Heather Gilbert, MS, OTR/L; and Michelle M. Rampulla, MS, OTR/L, CPRP

Mental Health in a Nutshell

Mental health occupational therapy practitioners focus on supporting people working toward their recovery. Although many definitions of *recovery* exist, most practitioners adopt the Substance Abuse and Mental Health Services Administration's (SAMHSA, 2012) definition: "a process of change through which individuals improve their health and wellness, live a self-directed life, and strive to reach their full potential" (p. 3). SAMHSA further defines the key components on which to focus when supporting people in recovery: health, home, purpose, and community. These focal points align well with occupational therapy's philosophy and practice, making therapists adept at helping clients during all stages of recovery.

Occupational Therapy's Role

A day in the life of a mental health occupational therapy practitioner varies depending on the setting, caseload, climate, and acuity of the milieu. Most therapists working in a mental health setting begin the day by communicating with the treatment team in meetings (in person or by phone) or by email. They organize their day around a combination of occupational therapy evaluations for new admissions, group prepping, occupational therapy treatment in both group and individual sessions, meeting with families, doing documentation, and performing other assessments as requested by physicians.

Akselrud, R. (Ed.). *Quintessential Occupational Therapy:*
A Guide to Areas of Practice (pp 95-104).
© 2023 Taylor & Francis Group.

TABLE 8-1

Common Diagnoses Treated by Occupational Therapists by Category

CATEGORY	DIAGNOSES AND COMMONLY USED ACRONYMS
Anxiety disorders	Generalized anxiety disorder (GAD), obsessive-compulsive disorder (OCD), post-traumatic stress disorder (PTSD), panic disorder
Mood disorders	Major depressive disorder (MDD), bipolar disorder
Psychotic disorders	Schizophrenia, delusional disorder, schizoaffective disorder, psychosis—not otherwise specified
Personality disorders	Borderline personality disorder, paranoid personality disorder, antisocial personality disorder
Neurocognitive disorders	Dementia, Alzheimer's disease, temporal-lobe dementia, vascular dementia, Korsakoff syndrome
Other disorders	Eating disorders, substance use disorders (SUD), dissociative disorders, autism spectrum disorder (ASD), intellectual and developmental disabilities

Commonly treated diagnoses include anxiety, mood, psychotic, personality, neurocognitive disorders, and substance use (Table 8-1). Often clients have a combination of psychiatric, cognitive, and medical issues that require occupational therapists to draw on their general knowledge in other areas, including addiction, transfer training, and home adaptations for aging clients with mobility or vision issues.

Numerous studies (Chang et al., 2011; Fok et al., 2012; Lawrence et al., 2010; Suetani et al., 2015) have determined that people living with serious mental illness experience a mortality rate higher than in the general population. According to Lawrence et al. (2010), the largest causes of death are cardiovascular and respiratory diseases. Various factors likely contribute to the lower life expectancy, including a higher rate of cigarette smoking, the lack of preventative care, time spent homeless or incarcerated, social isolation, low income, poor diet, substance abuse, and a sedentary lifestyle.

Occupational therapy can play a critical role in helping change lifestyles to reduce risk factors or manage chronic diseases. Mental health work can be rewarding for therapists who help clients through their struggle to build or rebuild their prior level of functioning or independence.

Caseload, Schedule, and Duties

The ratio of session types is dictated by agency or facility priorities. Caseload size depends on this ratio. Community-based mental health occupational therapists typically have a caseload of 20 to 25 clients. Those in hospital acute care settings may see 15 to 21 clients a day.

Full-time occupational therapists practicing in mental health work primarily weekday day shifts. Some settings may require evening, weekend, or holiday coverage. Part-time, per diem, and fee-for-service positions also may be available. Evaluation sessions vary by setting and may be 30, 60, or 90 minutes, depending on a client's ability to participate. Sometimes evaluations are completed over multiple shorter sessions. Treatment sessions may be 30, 45, or 60 minutes.

Occupational therapists attend the treatment team meetings and clinical reviews to aid in the development and implementation of individualized, patient-centered treatment plans. Additional duties include communicating with families, documenting in the medical record all evaluations performed and treatment provided, supervising fieldwork students, contributing to discharge planning, ordering sensory supplies, and providing training to other disciplines and direct-care staff.

Trauma

Occupational therapists treat the whole person and focus on increasing their ability to live as independently as possible in the least restrictive environment. Part of providing holistic care in a psychiatric setting is also being mindful of the impact of trauma. Research (Cusack et al., 2006; Mueser et al., 2004; Subica et al., 2012) has shown that 80% to 90% of people with mental health issues have experienced trauma. Therapists must understand the effects of trauma and be cautious not to retraumatize clients, as well as can play a critical role in the prevention of seclusion and restraint, last-resort strategies used when all other interventions have failed to keep a client from harming themselves or others. Efforts to de-escalate clients and teach them to use sensory modulation techniques to self-regulate are key to prevention of these potentially traumatizing strategies. Occupational therapists are uniquely qualified to address sensory processing and modulation challenges that result from trauma. Utilizing a sensory profile (Brown & Dunn, 2002) to identify and address sensory processing patterns that may be impacting occupational performance and/or ability to cope with the triggers associated with prior trauma. Sensory processing patterns can indicate hyposensitivity (disconnection with bodily senses) and hypersensitivity (activation of the autonomic nervous system or "fight or flight" response). Interventions which build skills in interoception can assist clients experiencing hypoarousal with building awareness of their body and the sensations related to various emotions as a precursor to emotional regulation (Mahler, 2015). Alternatively, a client whose autonomic nervous system is in hyperarousal may benefit from creating a sensory diet to modulate their system (Kimball, 2021). Both approaches allow clients to build insights and skills they can use to regulate their own responses to sensory stimuli, building self-efficacy and independence.

Medication Adherence, Coping Skills, and Self-Care

One of the most valuable skills occupational therapists have is to teach and educate clients recovering from mental illness about the importance of medication adherence and establishing coping skills. According to Bonder (2022), these components are at the forefront of most mental illnesses and later relapses. Many clients present in a facility with maladaptive behaviors (e.g., drinking, taking drugs, isolating, cutting and other self-injury, overeating, aggressiveness). Helping clients identify these behaviors and educating them about how to replace them with safer and more adaptive skills supports recovery (Bruce & Borg, 2015).

Although working in mental health can be emotionally taxing, the successes can provide fuel to keep going. Some successes are huge, such as seeing a client progress with improved schizophrenia symptoms from after a stay in jail and a recent suicide attempt to currently having a productive life that includes living independently, working part-time in the community, and caring for a pet. Even seemingly small successes are important, such as this example from an occupational therapist (H.H.) with more than 20 years experience in the field:

> Client X was a 53-year-old woman with major depression who attended my community reintegration group. The purpose of this group was for clients to set short-term goals (STGs) for themselves. Client X initially did not want to set STGs for herself because she stated, "What is the point? Every time I set goals for myself I don't accomplish them, and that makes me more depressed." Well, I convinced her to set the most concrete of STGs, ones related to self-care. Her goal was that she would shower at least four times within 1 week. The next morning on the unit, I saw Client X going to take shower, and she said, "One day down, three more

to go." This reaction did not stick with me as much as the reaction I saw when other clients noticed that Client X looked good after her shower and told her about it. The smile that Client X exhibited was the first one I had seen from her in her 2 weeks on the unit. The things that most of us take for granted are the things that we routinely do, like our self-care tasks. But for clients with mental illness, taking care of their self-care activities of daily living are often the first things they neglect.

Evaluation and Assessments

The initial evaluation uses a combination of a semi-structured interview to build an occupational profile (Figure 8-1), as well as functional observation and selected occupational therapy assessments, which can aid in developing an interdisciplinary treatment plan and determining the need for occupational therapy services (American Occupational Therapy Association, 2016). These assessments typically measure functional cognition, ability to perform activities of daily living or instrumental activities of daily living, or helping determine a client's valued roles and interests. Examples of commonly used assessments include the following:

- Mini-Mental State Exam
- Montreal Cognitive Assessment
- Allen Cognitive Level Screen
- Kohlman Evaluation of Living Skills
- Canadian Occupational Performance Measure
- Sensory Profile
- Sensory Processing Measure
- Occupational Circumstances Assessment Interview and Rating Scale
- Performance Assessment of Self-Care Skills
- Barth Time Construction
- Occupational Self-Assessment
- Stress Management Questionnaire
- Interests and Role Checklists
- Functional Independence Measure

Interventions

Occupational therapists working in mental health create an intervention plan in collaboration with clients and other team members, including social workers, nurses, psychologists, psychiatrists, health counselors, case managers, creative art therapists, nurse practitioners, nutritionists, and recreation therapists (Brown et al., 2011). Occupational therapy goals and interventions focus on skills development, community integration, and self regulation/emotional regulation.

Goals should be patient-centered and ideally in their own words (Table 8-2). Even unrealistic goals based in psychosis often can be used to create more beneficial or practical goals. Occupational therapists can help clients who for decades have had persistent delusions not treatable by medication or other strategies that work toward creating a reality orientation by using the delusions' theme to engage them in a conversation about goals (e.g., for a client believing they are an astronaut, encouraging them to take a sponge bath like astronauts do or to attend an art group by mentioning that they can create a blueprint for a rocket ship). Goal documentation varies by employer.

Occupational therapists use evidenced-based practices to improve clients' ability to self-regulate and participate in meaningful daily activities, including all areas of occupation, and increase independent living skills. Recovering meaningful roles, such as being a parent, may also be a focus of treatment.

Introduction

Hello, my name is _____. I am the occupational therapist here at _____. I would like to spend a little time with you to help me better understand who you are, why you are here, to tell you what my role is as a part of your treatment team, and to start thinking about how we can work together to reach your goals. It is okay if there are questions that you do not feel comfortable answering, just let me know that you do not wish to answer, and we can move on to the next one.

Questions to Consider Asking

- What is your name? What is today's date? Do you know where we are? (Orientation)
- What brought you here?
- Tell me about your living situation. Do you live in a private house, apartment, co-op, condominium, group home, or community facility? Do you live alone or with others?
- How do you get around? Do you drive or take public transportation?
- Who is in your social support system?
- Do you have any children?
- Do you have a job, or are you in school? Tell me about your work and educational history.
- Do you belong to any clubs or groups that you attend regularly?
- Do you have any hobbies, interests, or passions that bring you joy? If not, have you in the past?
- What was your typical day like before you came to the hospital?
- What was and still is important to you?
- What services are you currently receiving? Do you have a therapist? Are you taking any medication?
- Do you drink, do drugs, or smoke? If so, are you interested in stopping?
- What are your biggest stressors in life right now?
- What coping skills do you currently use?
- Where would you hope to go after you are discharged? (More specifically, what are your goals post-discharge?)

Explain what services you can provide for the client while they are in the facility and attending your program.

Figure 8-1. Sample occupational therapy initial interview.

Programming

Occupational therapists can help provide structure in the milieu of an inpatient unit, day program, or group living environment to promote client independence and support building healthy routines through a combination of environmental adaptations, staff training, group facilitation, and program development. Staff training can focus on recovery principles, sensory modulation basics, functional cognition, engagement strategies, client empowerment, and promotion of independence. Group interventions can include stress management, social skills, anger management, self-care, self-esteem, self-expression, healthy cooking, coping skills, life skills, sleep hygiene, medication adherence, and creative expression.

Reassessment and Discharge Planning

Mental health settings vary widely in length of stay or services; therefore, each setting will have its own requirements for frequency of reassessment. Reassessment may be utilized to justify continued occupational therapy services to assess changes in occupational performance, to update or set new goals, or to identify the level of support required upon discharge. Reassessment may also be

TABLE 8-2

Sample Client Goals in Mental Health

SETTING	EXAMPLES OF LONG-TERM GOALS	EXAMPLES OF SHORT-TERM GOALS	TARGETED OCCUPATIONS OR SKILLS
Community day program Length of participation can vary.	"I want to get and keep a job." Cindy will obtain and maintain part-time employment for at least 6 months.	Cindy will attend and participate in Job Club weekly. Cindy will help prepare and serve lunch in the kitchen unit at least three times per week. Cindy will identify and apply to at least one job per week with the assistance of staff. Cindy will identify and practice two sensory strategies she can use at work to self-regulate when hearing voices.	Vocational skills Food preparation Social skills Computer skills
Acute inpatient hospital Average length of stay is 3 days to 2 weeks.	"I need to learn how to deal with life." At discharge, Jim will independently identify stressors and articulate healthy coping mechanisms to use when triggers arise to prevent relapse.	Jim will attend three out of the five coping skills group sessions this week with moderate verbal cues or reminders to attend. Jim will identify four triggers that lead to stress by the end of the week with minimal assistance. Jim will identify four coping mechanisms to use when stressors arise by the end of the week with minimal assistance. Jim will participate in two leisure activities this week with moderate verbal cues or reminders to help him identify activities that he enjoys.	Trigger identification Stress management Coping skills Self-disclosure Time management Leisure

(continued)

TABLE 8-2 (CONTINUED)

Sample Client Goals in Mental Health

SETTING	EXAMPLES OF LONG-TERM GOALS	EXAMPLES OF SHORT-TERM GOALS	TARGETED OCCUPATIONS OR SKILLS
Inpatient state hospital Length of stay can vary widely; clients may stay weeks, months, or years.	"I want to build a rocket ship for when I go traveling." Mark will participate in social activities and unit groups at least three times per week within 3 months.	Mark will attend and participate in art group weekly with moderate cueing to build leisure and social skills. Mark will attend music and movement group weekly to learn a basic stretching routine he can complete while traveling. Mark will sponge bathe himself at least two times per week with moderate cueing and set-up.	Social interaction Physical activity Hygiene Leisure

used to gather additional information to inform an occupational profile if a client was not initially able to meaningfully participate in or tolerate the initial evaluation process (Brown et al., 2019). Important aspects to document during a reassessment include the need for skilled occupational therapy intervention, barriers to progress and how to address these, actual progress toward goals, functional outcomes, and client statements about how they feel occupational therapy has helped them. For clients who have met all their goals, who no longer wish to continue therapy, or who no longer need skilled therapy, occupational therapists will complete a treatment note and discharge summary. Discharge planning will also vary by setting, but generally includes providing a summary of the client's progress toward their goals, current functional status, and recommendations. The recommendations section might include suggestions for carry over of skills and/or strategies learned, relapse prevention strategies, connections to community groups or peer support specialists, and/or education for staff at the receiving facility or program of how to best support the client's continued progress.

Availability of Work

Occupational therapy positions in mental health may not be readily available in all areas. Busy metropolitan areas are more likely to have positions available while suburban or rural are less likely. Some occupational therapists elect to work in mental health in positions not specific to the profession (e.g., case managers, program directors). By showing occupational therapy's distinct value while holding such positions, therapists can advocate for new occupational therapy positions to be created within an agency or facility.

Compensation

Mental health occupational therapy salaries can fluctuate by source and year. According to the U.S. Bureau of Labor Statistics (2020) in 2019, the occupational therapy median salary in New York was $83,200, and in the same year the *Occupational Therapy Salary Guide* reported the annual salary as $76,448.

Per diem and fee-for-service positions pay more per hour than do full-time positions but usually offer no benefits. Full-time positions typically have benefits, such as paid time off and health insurance, but the salaries can be lower. State positions (e.g., inpatient state hospitals) may provide pensions.

Occupational therapists can be effective leaders and thus can earn higher salaries when taking on management positions. After significant experience in mental health, clinicians can apply to teach at the college level in their specialty.

Continuing Education

Occupational therapists entering mental health practice can benefit from reviewing or learning about cognitive-behavioral therapy, trauma-informed care, best practices for preventing seclusion and restraint (Huckshorn, 2006), sensory integration and modulation, motivational interviewing strategies, and effective group facilitation. Helpful frames of references to review include psychodynamic, behavioral, cognitive-behavioral therapy, cognitive disability, the Person–Environment–Occupation–Performance Model (Baum et al., 2015), the Model of Human Occupation (Kielhofner & Burke, 1980), and the Transtheoretical Model (or the Stages of Change; Prochaska et al., 2008). Interested students can seek a mental health fieldwork placement.

To better understand client diagnoses in this practice area, reviewing the latest editions of the *Diagnostic and Statistical Manual of Mental Disorders, Fifth Edition* (American Psychiatric Association, 2013) and the *International Classification of Diseases and Related Health Problems* (World Health Organization, 2019) is helpful. It also is useful to begin brainstorming individual and group treatment ideas. Having a thorough understanding of the HIPAA (Health Insurance Portability and Accountability Act of 1996) law is crucial for working with this population.

General Advice

The following are tips to help increase success in practice:
- Build work–life balance to allow time for self-care and engagement in activities and relationships that replenish energy and help avoid burnout because working with people who have experienced trauma can be difficult and draining.
- Break the stigma of mental health and educate about diseases and mental health work.
- Set firm boundaries in the workplace and with clients.
- Create a routine for success.
- Familiarize yourself with the work of Tina Champagne, Bessel van der Kolk, Brené Brown, Kelly Mahler, Albert Bandura, and others in the mental health field.
- Utilize resources available from the National Alliance on Mental Illness, Office of Minority Health, SAMHSA, and American Occupational Therapy Association, including information on evidence-based practices and guiding models.
- Consider working toward a certified psychiatric rehabilitation practitioner to create access to additional employment opportunities.
- Build awareness of personality traits and tendencies to build strong therapeutic relationships.

- Do not avoid difficult conversations, including those that involve risk assessment. Confront concerns (e.g., ask clients whether they have thoughts or a plan to harm themselves or another person, and if so, refer them to their physician, a crisis center, or the emergency department).

- Be mindful about professional boundaries. Do not share personal identifying information. Redirect intrusive questions by asking clients a question about themselves instead. Do not accept any gifts of value. Do not communicate with former clients once they have returned to the community—not by phone, mail, email, or social media.

- Consider emerging practice areas in mental health (e.g., forensics [treating clients involved with the criminal justice system], group living environments, day programs, homeless shelters or outreach teams, psychosocial clubhouses, supported employment, pediatric mental health).

- Seek opportunities when occupational therapy can solve a problem, and be bold when advocating for the profession's unique role and value. Get involved in agency workgroups or committees and contribute to initiatives (e.g., Zero Suicide).

Tips and Advice From the Field

Suitability for Practice

Thriving in the mental health field requires a combination of essential character traits and clinical knowledge. Clients recovering from serious mental illness and life traumas have dynamic needs, and due to the nature of their illnesses or history, may have challenges with trust, social relationships, or emotional regulation. Successful mental health occupational therapy practitioners should have patience, empathy, strong self-awareness and self-esteem, and the ability to stay calm in stressful situations, as well as be nonjudgmental, adaptable, creative, bold, and self-directed. It also is important to have a team mentality, to demonstrate a willingness to take initiative, and to have the ability to advocate for clients as well as for the value of occupational therapy.

In addition, occupational therapists may encounter clients who have been involved in the criminal justice system at some point in their lives. Most people with mental illness are not violent, but for some, symptoms, substance use, or trauma can lead to them demonstrating risky behaviors and, at times, getting into trouble with the law. Clinicians working in mental health should be able to accept that clients' worst behavior when symptomatic is not always representative of who they really are as people once they are stable with medication. Because clients may say hurtful things or become aggressive, it is crucial to have "thick skin" and use de-escalation techniques while not taking it personally.

References

American Occupational Therapy Association. (2016). *Occupational therapy's role in mental health recovery* [Fact sheet]. https://www.aota.org/-/media/Corporate/Files/AboutOT/Professionals/WhatIsOT/MH/Facts/Mental%20Health%20 Recovery.pdf

American Psychiatric Association. (2013). *Diagnostic and statistical manual of mental disorders* (5th ed.). https://doi.org/10.1176/appi.books.9780890425596

Baum, C. M., Christiansen, C. H., & Bass, J. D. (2015). The Person–Environment–Occupation–Performance (PEOP) model. In C. H. Christiansen, C. M. Baum, & J. D. Bass (Eds.), *Occupational therapy: Performance, participation, and well-being* (4th ed., pp. 49–56). SLACK Incorporated.

Bonder, B. R. (2022). *Psychopathology and function* (6th ed.). SLACK Incorporated.

Brown, C. E., & Dunn, W. (2002). *Adolescent/adult sensory profile*. Pearson.

Brown, C., Stoffel, V. C., & Munoz, J. P. (2011). *Occupational therapy in mental health: A vision for participation*. F. A. Davis.

Brown, C., Stoffel, V. C., & Munoz, J. (2019). *Occupational therapy in mental health: A vision for participation* (2nd ed.). F. A. Davis.

Bruce, M. A., & Borg, B. (2015). *Psychosocial frames of reference* (4th ed.). SLACK Incorporated.

Chang, C.-K., Hayes, R. D., Perera, G., Broadbent, M. T. M., Fernandes, A. C., Lee, W. E., Hotopf, M., & Stewart, R. (2011). Life expectancy at birth for people with serious mental illness and other major disorders from a secondary mental health care case register in London. *Plos One, 6*(5), e19590. https://doi.org/10.1371/journal.pone.0019590

Cusack, K. J., Grubaugh, A. L., Knapp, R. G., & Frueh, B. C. (2006). Unrecognized trauma and PTSD among public mental health consumers with chronic and severe mental illness. *Community Mental Health Journal, 42,* 487–500. https://doi.org/10.1007/s10597-006-9049-4

Fok, M. L.-Y., Hayes, R. D., Change, C.-K., Stewart, R., Callard, F. J., & Moran, P. (2012). Life expectancy at birth and all-cause mortality among people with personality disorder. *Journal of Psychosomatic Research, 73*(2), 104–107. https://doi.org/10.1016/j.jpsychores.2012.05.001

Health Insurance Portability and Accountability Act of 1996, Pub. L. No. 104-191, § 264, 110 Stat. 1936.

Huckshorn, K. A. (2006). *Six core strategies for reducing seclusion and restraint use.* National Association of State Mental Health Directors. https://www.nasmhpd.org/sites/default/files/Consolidated%20Six%20Core%20Strategies%20Document.pdf

Kielhofner, G., & Burke, J. P. (1980). A model of human occupation, part 1. Conceptual framework and content. *American Journal of Occupational Therapy, 34*(9), 572–581. https://doi.org/10.5014/ajot.34.9.572

Kimball, J. G. (2021). *Dial it down: A wellness approach for addressing post-traumatic stress in veterans, first responders, healthcare workers, and others in this uncertain world.* BookBaby.

Lawrence, D., Kisely, S., & Pais, J. (2010). The epidemiology of excess mortality in people with mental illness. *Canadian Journal of Psychiatry, 55*(12), 752–760. https://doi.org/10.1177/070674371005501202

Mahler, K. (2015) *Interoception: The eighth sensory system: Practical solutions for improving self-regulation, self-awareness and social understanding.* AAPC.

Mueser, K. T., Salyers, M. P., Rosenberg, S. D., Goodman, L. A., Essock, S. M., Osher, F. C., Swartz, M. S., Butterfield, M. I., & 5 Site Health and Risk Study Research Committee. (2004). Interpersonal trauma and posttraumatic stress disorder in patients with severe mental illness: Demographic, clinical, and health correlates. *Schizophrenia Bulletin, 30*(1), 45–57. https://doi.org/10.1093/oxfordjournals.schbul.a007067

Prochaska, J. O., Redding, C. A., & Evers, K. E. (2008). The transtheoretical model and stages of change. In K. Glanz, B. K. Rimer, & K. Viswanath (Eds.), *Health behavior and health education: Theory, research, and practice* (pp. 97–121). Jossey-Bass.

Subica, A. M., Claypoole, K. H., & Wylie, A. M. (2012). PTSD's mediation of the relationships between trauma, depression, substance abuse, mental health, and physical health in individuals with severe mental illness: Evaluating a comprehensive model. *Schizophrenia Research, 136*(1–3), 104–109. https://doi.org/10.1016/j.schres.2011.10.018

Substance Abuse and Mental Health Services Administration. (2012). *SAMHSA's working definition of recovery* [PDF]. https://store.samhsa.gov/system/files/pep12-recdef.pdf

Suetani, S., Whiteford, H. A., & McGrath, J. J. (2015). An urgent call to address the deadly consequences of serious mental disorders. *JAMA Psychiatry, 72*(12), 1166–1167. https://doi.org/10.1001/jamapsychiatry.2015.1981

U.S. Bureau of Labor Statistics. (2020, July 6). *Occupational employment and wages.* https://www.bls.gov/oes/2019/may/oes291122.htm

World Health Organization. (2019). *International classification of diseases* (11th rev.). https://icd.who.int/

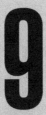

9

Outpatient Low Vision

*Yu-Pin Hsu, EdD, OTR/L; Inna Babaeva, PhD, OTR/L;
and AnneMarie O'Hearn, MEd, MPA*

Outpatient Low Vision in a Nutshell

Low vision is vision loss that cannot be corrected to normal with standard eyeglasses, contact lenses, and medical or surgical interventions. This loss of visual function can result from several disorders, frequently affecting patients' performance in activities of daily living (ADLs), such as reading, writing, and preparing meals. Even seemingly mild visual function loss can significantly affect visual tasks, particularly if comorbid conditions exist.

Vision rehabilitation is comprehensive, multidisciplinary care that helps patients with low vision maximize their residual vision and improve ADLs functioning. Services are provided by a range of professionals and may include a low vision evaluation, training in use of low vision devices, ADLs and instrumental activities of daily living (IADLs) rehabilitation, environmental modifications, travel training, and adaptive technology training.

Causes and Effects of Low Vision

Common causes of low vision include eye diseases, such as macular degeneration, glaucoma, diabetic retinopathy and retinitis pigmentosa, optic nerve damage, traumatic brain injury, and dystrophy of the eye's cones, rods, or macula. Other potential vision-threatening conditions include trauma to the eye, cancer, and genetic eye conditions.

While the impact on vision from these causes is unique to each patient, common visual impairments include loss of central visual field, loss of peripheral visual fields, blurry or distorted vision, or a combination of these. Patients with low vision also often experience loss of contrast sensitivity and increased sensitivity to light and glare (Figure 9-1).

Akselrud, R. (Ed.). *Quintessential Occupational Therapy:*
A Guide to Areas of Practice (pp 105-111).
© 2023 Taylor & Francis Group.

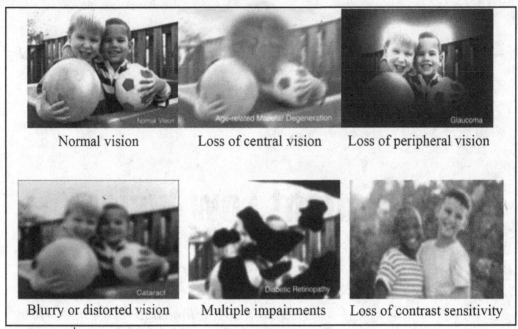

Normal vision   Loss of central vision   Loss of peripheral vision

Blurry or distorted vision   Multiple impairments   Loss of contrast sensitivity

Figure 9-1. Examples of low vision issues. (Reproduced with permission from National Eye Institute, National Institutes of Health.)

Occupational Therapy's Role

Occupational therapists are an integral part of the team providing rehabilitation services to patients with low vision. Therapists collaborate with optometrists, physical therapists, social workers, and low vision rehabilitation specialists (e.g., orientation and mobility instructors, teachers of those with visual impairments, adaptive technology specialists). This chapter discusses the role of occupational therapists treating adults in outpatient settings.

Low Vision in Outpatient Settings

In outpatient settings, occupational therapists identify vision problems and determine how low vision may be affecting patients' ADLs and IADLs. Therapists conduct basic vision assessments and use the findings, along with information about a patient's vision history, to formulate functional goals and interventions that address the identified impairments and improve patient occupational performance. In low vision clinics or vision rehabilitation agencies, therapists work closely with low vision physicians to determine the impact of vision loss on patient function, identify appropriate low vision devices, and develop interventions to address performance deficits.

Suitability for Practice

Low vision settings are generally fast paced, and patients require significant attention to address the physical and psychosocial effects of their vision loss. For the most part, experience in inpatient or outpatient settings is recommended before transitioning into a low vision position. In fact, most agencies require occupational therapists to have 3 to 5 years of experience before hiring them to provide specialized vision rehabilitation.

Problem

Client has no vision in their left eye and visual acuity of 20/400 in their right eye. They are unable to read their mail, write, safely pour a cup of hot liquid, and monitor their blood sugar and blood pressure.

Goals to Address Writing

(Similar goals will address reading, pouring skills, and monitoring blood sugar and blood pressure.)

- *Long-Term Goal:* Client will independently write a grocery list using compensatory print, bold, and space (PBS) technique before discharge (date).
- *Short-Term Goal 1:* Client will receive instruction in using PBS technique to write a list of several grocery items legibly in two sessions (date).
- *Short-Term Goal 2:* Client will write a grocery list legibly using PBS technique without verbal cueing and read back what they wrote in two sessions (date).

Figure 9-2. Sample occupational therapy goals for a patient with low vision.

Schedule and Caseload

In most outpatient agencies, occupational therapists have a 9:00 a.m. to 5:00 p.m. schedule with a lunch break. A typical caseload is five to seven patients per day, depending on whether the cases are new and on the length of the rehabilitation sessions. An initial evaluation or assessment is usually scheduled for 60 minutes, and treatment sessions range from 45 to 60 minutes. Patients will be scheduled for one to two sessions weekly or biweekly depending on their rehabilitation needs. Occupational therapists can also expect to spend about 1 hour per day in discussions with eye doctors, social workers, and other professionals involved in patient care or in talking with insurance providers.

Evaluation and Assessments

Occupational therapists use a variety of strategies and standardized and nonstandardized tools to determine patients' functional vision and formulate functional goals (Figure 9-2) and appropriate interventions to improve their occupational performance. Clinics may use their own version of a vision evaluation form (Table 9-1).

Therapists first develop a vision history through personal interview and a medical or eye chart review, which may include asking patients questions such as "Do you have trouble seeing well enough to read, cook, or feed yourself?" and observing if they squint, hold reading material close to their face, or bump into things when walking. When possible, therapists check medical records for eye diagnoses or references to a vision problem in the physician, nursing, or therapy notes.

Then occupational therapists conduct a basic vision assessment. Depending on patient diagnosis and identified functional limitations, therapists may assess near and intermediate visual acuity, reading speed and endurance, writing performance, visual fields, scotomas and preferred retinal locus, and contrast sensitivity.

Examples of commonly used standardized assessments include the following:

- *Canadian Occupational Performance Measure* (Law, 2019): Although not designed specifically for low vision, this tool provides outcome measurements that are useful for determining a patient's vision-related goals and formulating a treatment plan.
- *Early Treatment Diabetic Retinopathy Study Chart* (Shamir, 2015): This chart, which was designed for patients with low vision, has block, high-contrast letters; can measure visual acuity as low as 20/800; and can be used to test vision at 1, 2, and 4 meters.
- *Lighthouse game or number cards* (Lighthouse International, 2022): These cards test near visual acuity and habitual working distance.

TABLE 9-1

Typical Vision-Related Information on an Occupational Therapy Evaluation Form

Patient name, date of birth	Date
Eye diagnosis, ICD–10 codes	Referring doctor name and phone
Past medical history	Chief complaints
Other services patient is receiving	History of falls in past 6 months
Social/employment history	Any assistive devices for mobility
How patient travels to services	Sensorimotor screening
Vitals • Last blood sample/date • BP/HR at start of evaluation • BP/HR at end of evaluation	• Pain rating/type/contributing factors • UE AROM and muscle strength • UE sensation • Balance/equilibrium • Proprioception
ADLs/IADLs • Feeding • Bathing • Grooming • Dressing • Toileting • Dialing telephone • Ability to tell time • Pouring water • Communication skills • Medication management • Meal preparation • Financial management • Playing cards • Sewing • Clothing management • Community activities (shopping, travel) • Mobility • Ability to evacuate home in emergencies	Cognition and perception • Orientation to person, time, place, date • Ability to follow 2- and 3-step instructions • Insight and judgment • Problem solving • Right/left discrimination • Body part identification • Short-term memory
	Vision status • Last vision exam/Dr. • Last low vision exam/Dr./location • Glasses: distance/near/bifocals • Low vision devices/date of training • Visual acuity: distance/near • Dominant eye • Ocular alignment • Saccades • Tracking • Fixation • Reading assessment

(continued)

TABLE 9-1 (CONTINUED)

Typical Vision-Related Information on an Occupational Therapy Evaluation Form

Client goals	
	• Writing assessment
	• Visual field assessment observation/ confrontation
	• Contrast sensitivity function assessment
	• Glare/lighting symptoms
	• Filters indoors/outdoors
	• Color vision

ADLs = activities of daily living; AROM = active range of motion; BP/HR = blood pressure/heart rate; IADLs = instrumental activities of daily living; UE = upper extremity.

- *Pelli–Robson Chart* (Thayaparan et al., 2007): This chart, which measures contrast sensitivity, has rows of letters of the same size but with decreasing contrast that patients read until none can be seen.
- *Minnesota Low Vision Reading Acuity Chart* (Calabrèse et al., 2016): This chart assesses reading performance by measuring patients' reading acuity, critical print size, and maximum reading speed.
- *Pepper Test* (Watson et al., 1990): This assessment uses various reading print size charts to assess reading performance in adults with central scotomas.

Examples of less formal, nonstandardized strategies that are commonly used include the following:

- Assessing central fields for scotoma by having patients look straight ahead at a clock face and identify the numbers that are clearest and those that are blurry or missing.
- Assessing peripheral fields by the therapist holding their hands out to their sides and asking patients to identify the number of fingers being held up while maintaining their center gaze on the therapist's face.
- Assessing writing skills by asking for a demonstration.

Interventions

Assessment results are used to develop functional goals and treatment interventions that address how loss of vision is impacting a patient's function. For example, for patients with macular degeneration, central vision is most likely to be affected, and activities such as reading, writing, and recognizing faces may be difficult. Interventions may include reading skills exercises using an eccentric viewing position, preferred retinal locus training, exercises for writing skills, and environmental modifications (e.g., appropriate lighting, glare control, magnifiers, telescopes, electronic visual aids).

Patients with reduced peripheral visual field and possible depth perception problems as a result of glaucoma may have difficulty with ADLs such as finding items of clothing in the closet or food in the refrigerator and with safe mobility in unfamiliar or crowded environments. Interventions can include training in strategies to compensate for loss of visual field and depth perception, visual scanning training, and education on appropriate lighting and glare control.

Discharge Planning

Once clients achieve their rehabilitation goals, they are discharged from occupational therapy. A patient education program is included in the discharge plan to reinforce the use of low vision devices or assistive technology (e.g., magnifiers, electronic video magnifiers, other wearable visual devices) that may have been prescribed to assist in basic daily activities and instrumental activities, such as grooming, reading, writing, using a computer, watching television, and financial management. It may also include instructions to reinforce visual skills exercises, such as utilizing the better eye for scanning, fixation, pursuit, and saccades. Resources to access low vision applications and use accessibility features on smartphones and tablets may also be provided. After being discharged from occupational therapy, many clients receive other vision rehabilitation services that they may have been receiving simultaneously to occupational therapy, such as counseling and support services, orientation mobility instruction, career search and job placement services, and adaptive technology training.

Tips and Advice From the Field

Treating patients with low vision requires much patience and empathy, as well as good communication skills, including consistent use of descriptive language and verbal cues while at the same time working in a fast-paced environment. Patients are often dealing with a range of emotions related to losing their vision and may easily become frustrated or angry. Setting personal boundaries may be necessary.

Before entering vision rehabilitation, occupational therapy practitioners should take low vision continuing education courses and review articles and textbooks on low vision diagnoses as well as their impact on functional vision. This work is needed to learn how to interpret eye exams and vision assessments. It can also be beneficial to find an occupational therapy mentor with experience treating patients with low vision. Therapists who desire to enter the field must be independent self-learners with a commitment to keep up with the current literature, treatment options, and rapidly advancing technology for patients with low vision impairments.

Resources for Low Vision

- *Home Lighting Assessment for Clients With Low Vision* (Perlmutter et al., 2013)
- *Low Vision Rehabilitation: A Practical Guide for Occupational Therapists* (Scheiman et al., 2007)
- *Occupational Therapy Interventions for Older Adults With Low Vision* (Beckley, 2016)
- *Occupational Therapy Interventions to Improve the Reading Ability of Older Adults With Low Vision: A Systematic Review* (Smallfield et al., 2013)

References

Beckley, M. N. (2016). Occupational therapy interventions for older adults with low vision. In K. Barney & M. Perkinson (Eds.), *Occupational therapy with aging adults: Promoting quality of life through collaborative practice* (pp. 155–167). Elsevier.

Calabrèse, A., Owsley, C., McGwin, G., & Legge, G. E. (2016). Development of a reading accessibility index using the MNREAD Acuity Chart. *JAMA Ophthalmology, 134*(4), 398-405. https://doi.org/10.1001/jamaophthalmol.2015.6097

Law, M., Baptiste, S., Carswell, A., McColl, M. A., Polatajko, H. J., & Pollock, N. (2019). *Canadian Occupational Performance Measure* (5th ed.). http://www.thecopm.ca/

Lighthouse International. (2022). *PowerCard number & word recognition pocket-size test card.* https://www.bernell.com/product/USOLPC/Assessments_New

National Eye Institute. (2022). *NEI media library.* https://medialibrary.nei.nih.gov/

Perlmutter, M. S., Bhorade, A., Gordon, M., Hollingsworth, H., Engsberg, J. E., & Baum, M. C. (2013). Home lighting assessment for clients with low vision. *American Journal of Occupational Therapy, 67*(6), 674–682. https://doi.org/10.5014/ajot.2013.006692

Scheiman, M., Scheiman, M., & Whittaker, S. G. (2007). *Low vision rehabilitation: A practical guide for occupational therapists*. SLACK Incorporated.

Shamir, R. R., Friedman, Y., Joskowicz, L., Mimouni, M., & Blumenthal, E. Z. (2015). Comparison of Snellen and Early Treatment Diabetic Retinopathy Study charts using a computer simulation. *International Journal of Ophthalmology, 9*(1), 119–123. https://doi.org/10.18240/ijo.2016.01.20

Smallfield, S., Clem, K., & Myers, A. (2013). Occupational therapy interventions to improve the reading ability of older adults with low vision: A systematic review. *American Journal of Occupational Therapy, 67*(3), 288–295. https://doi.org/10.5014/ajot.2013.004929

Thayaparan, K., Crossland, M. D., & Rubin, G. S. (2007). Clinical assessment of two new contrast sensitivity charts. *The British Journal of Ophthalmology, 91*(6), 749–752. https://doi.org/10.1136/bjo.2006.109280

Watson, G. R., Baldasare, J., & Whittaker, S. (1990). The validity and clinical uses of the Pepper Visual Skills for Reading Test. *Journal of Visual Impairment & Blindness, 84*(3), 119–123. https://doi.org/10.1177/0145482X9008400304

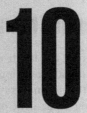

10

Assistive Technology

Rachelle Lydell, MSOT, OTR/L
and Douglene Jackson, PhD, OTR/L, LMT, ATP, CYT, FAOTA

Assistive Technology in a Nutshell

Assistive technology includes devices, services, strategies, and practices that are conceived and applied to ameliorate the functional challenges of individuals with disabilities or impairments (Assistive Technology Act of 2004; World Health Organization, 2022). Occupational therapy practitioners can provide assistive technology services, including assessments, device creation and modifications, recommendations, and interventions, to improve patients' functional performance and participation.

Occupational therapists can incorporate assistive technology into everyday professional practice, work as part of an interdisciplinary team, or be employed part-time or full-time in specialty programs within hospitals, schools, clinics, universities, governmental organizations, or other community-based settings. In addition, therapists can advocate for equitable access to assistive technology to foster occupational performance and participation domestically and internationally (World Federation of Occupational Therapists, 2022).

Several interprofessional models and frameworks are used to guide assistive technology practice. One of the most widely used is Cook et al.'s (1995) Human Activity Assistive Technology, which involves a patient engaging in an activity using assistive technology within their environment. Zalaba (1995) has proposed the Student, Environment, Tasks, and Tools Framework, which is used primarily in educational settings and has expanded to other contexts. Scherer (2002) has created the Matching Person and Technology Model, which consists of person-centered assessment measures for personal strengths, needs, preferences, and perceived assistive technology benefits. Using these assistive technology approaches, occupational therapists can work individually or collaboratively to improve patient quality of life.

Akselrud, R. (Ed.). *Quintessential Occupational Therapy:*
A Guide to Areas of Practice (pp 113-122).
© 2023 Taylor & Francis Group.

Occupational Therapy's Role

Occupational therapy practitioners are at the assistive technology forefront, collaborating with patients and other health professionals to make decisions about assistive technology use, as well as utilizing their skills to fabricate assistive technology using low- and high-technology means. Through simple modifications to existing equipment or using various materials, including 3D printing, therapists can contribute to assistive technology customization and creation (Aflatoony & Shenai, 2021). In addition, various organizations promote collaboration with others to increase equitable access to assistive technology and free and low-cost means for creation, including AT Makers (www.atmakers.org) and Makers Making Change (www.makersmakingchange.com).

Occupational therapists can recommend assistive technology for individuals with disabilities or who are experiencing challenges with occupational performance at any stage of life. For example, in early childhood, patients might benefit from using adapted tools for feeding and drawing, modified controllers for video games, and augmentative and alternative communication (AAC) to promote social participation. In adulthood, patients might use assistive technology to perform self-care skills, support performance of work tasks, engage in driving, or participate in leisure activities. The overall goal is to consider the occupations that can be enhanced using assistive technology and support patients in making informed decisions during product selection.

Sample Practice Setting:
Outpatient Adult and Pediatric Wheelchair Clinic

In an outpatient wheelchair specialty clinic, patients with qualifying diagnoses or mobility deficits can access a team of experts who work collaboratively to obtain specific equipment to increase participation in activities of daily living (ADLs). Full-service specialty clinics are rare; therefore, these clinics often are scheduled weekly, monthly, or as needed, depending on the resources available in that setting.

A wheelchair clinic in high demand is usually the result of a well-orchestrated collaboration among local primary care physicians, a local or national vendor, an assistive technology professional (ATP), and an evaluating occupational therapist who has a specialty background in assistive technology and complex rehabilitation technology. Some occupational therapists may be certified ATPs and also seating and mobility specialists.

In most cases, an ATP from a national or local supplier will be part of the team, with the primary role of assisting patients when acquiring the equipment from a vendor and facilitating third-party payment. One benefit of attending a wheelchair clinic for acquiring specialized assistive technology, such as power wheelchairs or scooters, is that national vendors often house mobility equipment, seating technology, and accessories at the evaluation site for patients to trial, which allows the team to effectively and efficiently evaluate, fit, and prescribe the appropriate equipment while reducing potential barriers and wait times for the equipment to be processed, ordered, and delivered for patient fitting, training, and eventual personal use.

For the provision of wheelchair services to occur, patients must have a mobility deficit despite the use of a cane, walker, or manual wheelchair; a health condition that impairs their ability to complete routine ADLs; the cognitive ability to operate a power mobility device (PMD); and the ability to safely transfer on and off the device with or without assistance. This initial assessment of eligibility is completed at a face-to-face meeting with the patient's primary care physician and is crucial for providing clinical guidance to not only the prescribing physician but also to the treating clinician for establishing medical necessity for the equipment. Once the physician certifies that the equipment is medically necessary, a written order is forwarded to the wheelchair clinic so that the team can complete a comprehensive patient evaluation, conduct a wheelchair assessment and trial, and prescribe the appropriate equipment.

Evaluations are typically scheduled during regular clinic hours or at specific times of day. In the latter case, this scheduling can allow time for the team to complete the required documentation and paperwork, which can be extensive depending on a patient's insurance coverage (e.g., Medicaid, Medicare, private insurance). A comprehensive wheelchair evaluation can take 2 to 3 hours to complete.

The specialty clinic team usually includes the evaluating occupational therapist and ATP. At times, a sales representative from a particular seller or vendor may be asked to be present, usually to provide the team with specific equipment for a patient to try and to allow the team, in collaboration with the patient and their family, to determine if the equipment is the right fit.

Occupational therapy practitioners are an important part of the assistive technology interdisciplinary team in the clinic. The team is critical to obtaining equipment because no one individual can meet all of the needs of service delivery. Every role in the process requires extensive collaboration with the patient, their family members, and other professionals.

Schedule and Caseload

The caseloads of occupational therapists working in a specialty clinic varies by setting. For example, an assistive technology clinic held once a week from 7:30 a.m. to 5:30 p.m. may schedule three to four patients if 2 to 3 hours are required for a comprehensive evaluation. Documentation time to write the occupational therapy evaluation and a letter of medical necessity may be scheduled as part of the 2- to 3-hour evaluation time slot depending on the setting.

A typical assistive technology caseload consists of patients scheduled for occupational therapy evaluations, assistive technology assessments, and equipment management and training sessions. A caseload also can include the procurement, management, and training in AAC devices, cognitive aids, computer access, electronic aids to daily living, sensory-integrative devices, seating and mobility, recreational equipment, environmental modifications, accessible transportation (public and private), and other technologies for children and adults with learning disabilities.

Evaluation and Assessments

The process and procedure of a typical wheelchair evaluation and the corresponding roles and responsibilities of each team member involved are outlined in Table 10-1.

During the occupational therapy evaluation, short-term goals are written to be completed at the end of the session. The following goals are examples of short-term goals written in the SMART (*s*pecific, *m*easurable, *a*chievable, *r*elevant, *t*ime-based) format for an occupational therapy evaluation completed for a patient needing a power wheelchair:

- Patient will be independent with relieving pressure in the wheelchair by week 2.
- Patient will demonstrate the ability to safely transfer in and out of the wheelchair by week 4.
- Patient will demonstrate independent mobility within the clinical environment to prepare for independence with mobility-related ADLs in two of three opportunities.
- Patient will demonstrate competency with operation and maneuvering of the wheelchair within the clinical environment to prepare for independence with mobility-related ADLs.

Tips and Advice From the Field

Occupational therapists with knowledge and an interest in assistive technology can work and apply their skills in traditional or nontraditional settings with patients of all ages with varying diagnoses. In traditional health care settings (e.g., outpatient or private practice clinics), therapists assess and prescribe mobility equipment and other assistive technology to patients as members of the interprofessional team. Therapists assist with the provision of adaptive dressing and feeding equipment, work in collaboration with speech–language pathologists to prescribe AAC, and consult

TABLE 10-1

Process and Procedures of a Typical Wheelchair Evaluation

ASSISTIVE TECHNOLOGY SERVICE DELIVERY PROCEDURE	TEAM MEMBER	ROLE AND RESPONSIBILITIES
Initial face-to-face appointment to discuss assistive technology need	Primary care physician	• Conducts a face-to-face examination of patient • Writes a prescription for a PMD with qualifying diagnosis, PMD description, conditions PMD is expected to modify, and signature and date of face-to-face examination • Forwards prescription to wheelchair clinic and/or treating therapist within 45 days of written prescription; may also forward to supplier
Occupational therapy evaluation	Occupational therapist	• Completes patient evaluation, including history and relevant review of systems, using pertinent physical assessments, tests, or measurements • Identifies targeted impaired patient performance areas, assesses functional needs, determines medical necessity for PMD (may include a functional capacity wheeled mobility evaluation) • Identifies patient goals, accounting for possible future needs • Completes all evaluation documentation (must state reason for initial referral to occupational therapy) • Completes billing procedures
Assistive technology assessment, including assistive technology trial and prescription	Occupational therapist	• Identifies and selects appropriate PMD • Plans and applies appropriate adaptations pertaining to increasing functional independence within a performance area • Assesses environmental, physical, and social contexts pertaining to potential use of PMD • Evaluates tasks, functional demands, and resources within environments

(continued)

TABLE 10-1 (CONTINUED)

Process and Procedures of a Typical Wheelchair Evaluation

ASSISTIVE TECHNOLOGY SERVICE DELIVERY PROCEDURE	TEAM MEMBER	ROLE AND RESPONSIBILITIES
	ATP	• Ensures safety during equipment trial and that PMD meets patient needs • Considers need for accessories, ergonomic factors, seating position, and sheerness when planning for increasing functional participation in daily routines • Completes the letter of medical necessity to justify PMD and all needed specifications • Evaluates patient needs in collaboration with treating therapist • Interprets patient evaluation results to determine how abilities relate to assistive technology use
	Primary care physician	• Assists with selection of appropriate PMD, provides technical-related assistance and training in use • Facilitates third-party payer processes and patient billing as the direct-to-consumer service • Receives wheelchair evaluation and letter of medical necessity • Signs documentation to support assistive technology prescription
Wheelchair management and training	Occupational therapist	• Ensures PMD arrives according to parameters specified during assessment • Trains patients to promote optimal safety, mobility, and transfers using skilled instruction on positioning, positioning supplies, prevention of decubitus ulcers, contractures, and other medical complications
	ATP	• Evaluates outcomes • Delivers selected PMD • Provides technical-related assistance and training in use

(continued)

TABLE 10-1 (CONTINUED)

Process and Procedures of a Typical Wheelchair Evaluation

ASSISTIVE TECHNOLOGY SERVICE DELIVERY PROCEDURE	TEAM MEMBER	ROLES AND RESPONSIBILITIES
Wheelchair management and training follow-up appointments	Occupational therapist	• May need three to four sessions for patient or caregiver training • Performs reevaluation as necessary, wheelchair modification, propulsion training, and energy conservation training

For more information on the process and flow for obtaining a PMD, see the Medicare Learning Network, https://www.cms.gov/outreach-and-education/medicare-learning-network-mln/mlngeninfo and Medicare Coverage for Mobility Assistive Equipment, http://www.cms.hhs.gov/CoverageGenInfo/06_wheelchair.asp. For more information on the ATP certification, see https://www.resna.org/Certification/Assistive-Technology-Professional-ATP.

with physical therapists to prescribe PMDs. It is important that despite the use of technology, the client-centered focus of occupational therapy practice remain (American Occupational Therapy Association [AOTA], 2016). Occupational therapists should focus on the client, the occupation, and the environment and context when choosing and designing assistive technology interventions (AOTA, 2016). Occupational therapists must decide when the assistive technology process requires the additional input of other personnel and/or more training.

Resources and Continuing Education

Many resources and learning opportunities exist in assistive technology, and occupational therapists should take advantage of these (Table 10-2).

Collaboration With Other Disciplines

In the private sector, occupational therapists can work as ATPs for a national seating and mobility company or vendor. In this role, therapists' knowledge of the human body and positioning strategies to enable functional participation, prevent further injury, and avoid decline in function make them crucial members of assistive technology teams. Therapists are skilled in the assessment of patients' needs and in identifying, selecting, and prescribing appropriate, practical equipment. Working in collaboration with a community provider or treating therapist (occupational or physical), ATPs can facilitate the provision of adaptive seating, feeding, mobility, or durable medical equipment necessary for increasing functional participation in ADLs through vendor processing, third-party billing, and technical knowledge and assistance.

In a school-based setting, assistive technology is an important part of the support system for students with a disability to gain access to the curriculum. The Individuals with Disabilities Education Act (2004) defines assistive technology as any "item, piece of equipment, or product system, whether acquired commercially off the shelf, modified, or customized, that is used to increase, maintain, or improve functional capabilities of a child with a disability" [20 U.S.C. §1401(1)(2) and 34 C.F.R. §300.5].

Table 10-2

Assistive Technology Resources and Education for Occupational Therapists

FACT SHEET AND OFFICIAL DOCUMENTS

- *Occupational Therapy's Role with Providing Assistive Technology Devices and Services* (AOTA, 2015)
- *Assistive Technology and Occupational Performance: AOTA Official Document* (AOTA, 2016)
- *Position Statement: Occupational Therapy and Assistive Technology* (World Federation of Occupational Therapists, 2019)

ASSOCIATIONS, NETWORKS, AND GROUPS

- Assistive Technology Industry Association: www.atia.org
- AT Makers: www.atmakers.org
- Job Accommodation Network: www.askjan.org
- Makers Making Change: www.makersmakingchange.com
- Quality Indicators for Assistive Technology Services: www.qiat.org
- Rehabilitation Engineering and Assistive Technology Society of North America: www.resna.org
- Student, Environment, Tasks, and Tools Framework: www.joyzabala.com

STATE AND FEDERALLY FUNDED PUBLIC HEALTH PROGRAMS

- TRIAD Program: https://www.justicecenter.ny.gov/traid-program
- Wisconsin's Assistive Technology Program: https://www.dhs.wisconsin.gov/disabilities/wistech/index.htm
- North Carolina Assistive Technology Program: https://www.ncdhhs.gov/divisions/vocational-rehabilitation-services/north-carolina-assistive-technology-program
- Illinois Assistive Technology Program: https://www.iltech.org/

ONLINE COURSES

- AOTA Online Course: Understanding the Assistive Technology Process to Promote School-Based Occupation Outcomes, presented by Beth Goodrich, MS, MEd, OTR, ATP; Lynn Gitlow, PhD, OTR/L, ATP; and Judith Schoonover, MEd, OTR/L, ATP: https://research.aota.org/ajot/article/67/1/126/5737/Continuing-Education
- The Assistive Technology Industry Association's Learning Center offers a number of courses found at: https://www.atia.org/path-lms/?pathPage=%2Fatia%2F
- Occupationaltherapy.com offers several assistive technology courses including:
  - Home Assessment and Modifications for Aging in Place: https://www.occupationaltherapy.com/ot-ceus/course/home-assessment-and-modifications-for-5663/
  - Assistive Technology Assessment and Service Delivery: Preparing for the ATP Exam: https://www.occupationaltherapy.com/ot-ceus/course/assessment-and-service-delivery-preparing-5547

(continued)

TABLE 10-2 (CONTINUED)

Assistive Technology Resources and Education for Occupational Therapists

- ° Assistive Technology Access: Preparing for the ATP Exam: https://www.occupationaltherapy.com/ot-ceus/course/assistive-technology-access-preparing-for-5542
- ° Occupational Therapy for Driving and Adaptive Equipment: https://www.occupationaltherapy.com/ot-ceus/course/occupational-therapy-for-driving-and-5504
- ° Assistive Technology and Environmental Modifications: https://www.occupationaltherapy.com/ot-ceus/assistive-technology-and-environmental-modifications/?utm_medium=cpc&gclid=Cj0KCQjwlK-WBhDjARIsAO2sErQeP_8TK3pvv2--e-dGlfkqdJGdnDk8MOol4zHJ8crnfBJ0ZWK5qGAaAkqFEALw_wcB

BLOG POST

- • "How to Get a Medicare-Covered Power Scooter or Wheelchair" by Jim T. Miller: https://www.huffpost.com/entry/how-to-get-a-medicare-cov_b_5698171

In this setting, occupational therapists are an important part of the Individualized Education Program team when making decisions about what is appropriate for a student receiving special-education–related services. Occupational therapists observe, implement, and evaluate specific skill sets in sensory, physical, and cognitive areas. In addition, therapists can address underlying skills required for effective assistive technology use, increase access, customize features, and implement methods for training the child, school staff, and family in device use and care.

In a public health setting, patients and families needing adaptive feeding, seating, or mobility devices that enable participation in daily routines must work in collaboration with other therapists, service coordinators, nurses, and case workers to follow state regulatory guidelines for assistive technology service provision. For example, occupational therapists working in early intervention or in an adult developmental disabilities residential program can coordinate the assistive technology loan closet process and procedures to ensure the timely provision of assistive technology to enable participation in daily routines or ensure continued independence with ADLs completion because loan closets in these settings typically act as a temporary solution for families with assistive technology needs until permanent equipment can be acquired.

In addition, public health programs that are state and federally funded that are designed to meet the Assistive Technology Act of 2004 provide assistive technology services, such as device demonstration, short-term device loans, and assistive technology reutilization. Examples of these programs include the North Carolina Assistive Technology Program, Illinois Assistive Technology Program, WisTech (Wisconsin), and TRIAD Program (New York State).

Suitability for Practice

Assistive technology is an interdisciplinary field, consisting of therapists, educators, engineers, and other professionals seeking to improve quality of life through assistive devices and services. As assistive technology service providers, occupational therapists can seek specialty certification to acknowledge their expertise. Certification as an ATP or seating and mobility specialist can be obtained through the Rehabilitation and Engineering Society of North America. A specialized certificate can also be obtained from completing coursework at higher education institutions.

Professional development and networking are key to remain current in assistive technology advances, with many conferences being dedicated toward those at various skill levels. Occupational therapists in assistive technology must proactively seek lifelong learning. The following groups have conferences that provide opportunities to learn and gain experience with creating assistive technology: the Assistive Technology Industry Association, the CSUN Assistive Technology Conference, Rehabilitation Engineering and Assistive Technology Society of North America, Closing the Gap, and the Assistive Technology Makers' Fair Conference and Expo.

Assistive technology is a specialty area of practice. Occupational therapy clinicians who have an interest in assistive technology may seek additional training to obtain the essential knowledge required in this area; however, mentoring from experienced clinicians is the best way to learn what knowledge and skills are necessary to be competent practitioners in this area. New occupational therapy graduates are advised to develop their knowledge base and foundational clinical skills before pursuing exclusive practice in assistive technology.

Letter of Medical Necessity

A letter of medical necessity is used for medical insurance companies to justify the need for medical equipment (Figure 10-1). Occupational therapists must produce a letter stating patient needs and why they require the recommended equipment. Therapists work closely with medical equipment companies to create this letter based on the availability and measurements that best fit a patient.

References

Aflatoony, L., & Shenai, S. (2021). Unpacking the challenges and future of assistive technology adaptation by occupational therapists. In *CHItaly, 14th Biannual Conference of the Italian SIGCHI Chapter* (pp. 1-8).

American Occupational Therapy Association. (2015). *Occupational therapy's role with providing assistive technology devices and services* [Fact sheet]. https://www.aota.org/-/media/corporate/files/aboutot/professionals/whatisot/rdp/facts/at-fact-sheet.pdf

American Occupational Therapy Association. (2016). Assistive technology and occupational performance. *American Journal of Occupational Therapy, 70*(Suppl. 2), 7012410030p1–7012410030p9. https://doi.org/10.5014/ajot.2016.706S02

Assistive Technology Act of 2004. 105 U.S.C. § 2432.

Cook, A. M., Polgar, J. M., & Hussey, S. M. (2008). *Cook & Hussey's human activity assistive technologies: Principles and practice.* Elsevier.

Individuals with Disabilities Education Act, 20 U.S.C § 1400 (2004).

Scherer, M. J. (Ed.). (2002). *Assistive technology: Matching device and consumer for successful rehabilitation.* American Psychological Association. https://doi.org/10.1037/10420-000

World Federation of Occupational Therapists. (2019). *Position statement: Occupational therapy and assistive technology.* https://wfot.org/resources/occupational-therapy-and-assistive-technology

World Federation of Occupational Therapists. (2022). *Welcome to the World Federation of Occupational Therapists.* https://www.wfot.org

World Health Organization. (2022). *World Health Organization.* https://www.who.int/home/search?indexCatalogue=genericsearchindex1&searchQuery=assistive%20device&wordsMode=AllWords

Zabala, J. S. (1995). The Sett Framework: A model for selection and use of assistive technology tools and more. *Assistive Technology to Support Inclusive Education,* 17–36. https://doi.org/10.1108/s1479-363620200000014005

Date:
Name of child:
Date of birth:
To Whom It May Concern:

(*Patient name*) is a (*positive adjective*) (#)-year-old (*boy or girl, man or woman*) with a diagnosis of (*list diagnosis[es]*). (*Describe patient general health condition.*) (*Describe patient impairments in structure and function.*) (*Describe patient functional abilities and impairments.*) (*Describe participatory-level routines, tasks, and activities that a patient does.*) Because of the aforementioned limitations and impairments (*patient name*) is unable to (*describe primary functional impairment*).

When (*patient name*) trialed the (**specific assistive technology device**), *they were* able to (*describe desired functional ability and its qualities: independently, distance, more efficiently, safely, etc.*). The (**specific assistive technology device**) with the following accessories will improve (*patient name*)'s independence and support their participation in (*describe routine, task, or activity*).

- **Extensor Assist Pad:** The Extensor Assist Pad is needed to improve (*patient name*)'s alignment in the sagittal plane. Without the Extensor Assist Pad, (*patient name*) will demonstrate persistent excessive hip flexion while walking. This is inefficient and puts (*them*) at risk of increased shortening of the hip flexors, and, potentially, further disintegration of (*their*) walking ability.
- **Pelvic Stabilizer:** The Pelvic Stabilizer supports the alignment of the user in the frontal plane. (*Patient name*) has a tendency to be asymmetric in (*their*) hip and spine (*statically, dynamically, in which positions?*). The Pelvic Stabilizer provides boundaries that will improve (*patient name*)'s pelvic symmetry in the frontal plane.
- **Forearm Supports:** Forearm supports are helpful when a person is unable to appropriately bear weight through one or both upper extremities. (*Patient name*) will need (*unilateral/bilateral*) forearm supports because (*they are*) unable to bear weight, through (*their*) upper extremities in alignment because (*why?*). Having the forearm supports on the gait trainer allows (*patient name*) to have improved alignment throughout (*their*) body, to bear weight through the upper extremities with improved alignment, and to optimize the overall efficiency of (*patient name*)'s gait.
- **Accessory A:** *Describe medical justification.*
- **Accessory B:** *Describe medical justification.*
- **Accessory C:** *Describe medical justification.*
- **Accessory D:** *Describe medical justification.*

Equipment Accessories/Enhancements
- **All-Terrain Wheel Kit:** All-Terrain Wheels are necessary to allow (*patient name*) to traverse over the uneven ground that (*they*) encounter at (*location*). Without the All-Terrain Wheels, (*patient name*) will be unable to fully participate in the environments in which (*they*) typically do.
- **Accessory/Enhancement A:** *Describe medical justification.*
- **Accessory/Enhancement B:** *Describe medical justification.*
- **Accessory/Enhancement C:** *Describe medical justification.*

In summary, (*patient name*) is unable to safely and effectively ambulate in (*environments patient is unable to walk in without the gait trainer*). The (**specific assistive technology device**) with the aforementioned accessories is the best choice for increasing (*patient name*)'s independence while maintaining (*their*) safety.

Your prompt attention to (*patient name*)'s needs is appreciated. Please feel free to contact me with any questions or for clarifications.

Professionally,
(*Occupational therapist's name and credentials*)
(*Contact information*)

Figure 10-1. Sample template for a letter of medical necessity for assistive technology and durable medical equipment.

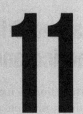

Academic Education

Ivelisse Lazzarini, EdD, OTD, OTR/L
and Gioia J. Ciani, MS, OTD, OTR/L

Academic Education in a Nutshell

Professional practicing occupational therapists are needed to enter academic education to help prepare future clinicians. This chapter discusses fundamental issues to consider when moving from an expert clinician's role to a novice academic role.

A higher education position involves the pursuit of knowledge and its dissemination and application through activities, such as teaching, service, research, publishing, and formal and informal professional presentations in areas of expertise. Critical to a faculty position is service that is congruent with the institutional mission and vision. Faculty can contribute through governance, educator associations, internal and external committees, community engagement, and state and national associations. These necessary activities involve aspects of teaching in an academic institution.

Higher education relies on active engagement in critical inquiry and research, both of which can inform the teaching and learning mission of institutions and are essential to developing society. All faculty must develop and maintain their academic competence and effectiveness to be proficient in their academic duties. Nonscheduled and scheduled activities require a balance to afford faculty adequate opportunity to participate in all academic work areas.

Transitioning from clinical practice to academic education involves professional and personal considerations. Academia and clinical practice are distinctly separate fields of expertise. Instead of patients, the target population in academia is students, whose needs and desires are different. Furthermore, although education is an essential component of competent occupational therapy practice, clinical expertise does not correspond to competency in the academic world.

Akselrud, R. (Ed.). *Quintessential Occupational Therapy:*
A Guide to Areas of Practice (pp 123-134).
© 2023 Taylor & Francis Group.

Similarities and Differences Between Practice and Education

Occupational therapists may consider transitioning into academia because of supposedly working fewer and more flexible hours. Two of the most popular reasons for transitioning to a career in academia are desire and preference for teaching and a desire to share clinical knowledge and experiences (Vassantachart & Rice, 1997). Therapists report feeling increasingly pressured to do more with less—to see more patients with complex diagnoses in less time and with fewer supports—and have little time to discuss patients with colleagues, to reflect on treatment strategies, or to make safe placements.

Occupational therapists in most clinical practices may be used to days booked with patients scheduled every 30 to 45 minutes and two short lunch breaks. In comparison, occupational therapy faculty calendars may look *empty*, with two to three scheduled courses to teach in a week, along with committee meetings, office hours, and student appointments. Therefore, it is reasonable for clinicians to ponder what faculty do all day.

Faculty members are likely to answer that they are busier than ever—usually referring to academia as a career and not just a job with structured hours that can be left behind at the end of the day or week. Frequently, faculty report feeling overwhelmed by increasing student needs, grading exams and papers, and developing and grading course competencies. Preparing lectures requires time to research current evidence for an increasing number of complex rehabilitation problems. Adaptations to teaching styles and different theoretical approaches to education may be required to better fit the needs of today's students, who may be learning in a traditional classroom or from an online platform using a learning management system.

Although both roles require considerable energy and a commitment to excellence, the decision to seek an academic role should prompt clinicians to assess and reflect on their preferred work environment and skill set. Does one like the constant stimulation and feedback of clinical practice? Does one enjoy days that fly by, surrounded by colleagues and patients, moving from one case to another, engaging socially and professionally, knowing that one has made a difference in patients' or colleagues' lives? Occupational therapists who best adapt to a faculty role are likely to have strong interpersonal skills, are self-starting and self-directed, do not rely heavily on directions from others, and do not mind spending time alone researching, editing, and writing. Whereas this work sounds delightful to some, losing patient contact may be an issue for others.

Both academic and clinical occupational therapists can make significant and lifelong contributions to health care. When providing rehabilitation services for patients, the impact is immediate and obvious. Education's rewards are less direct and require confidence that one's students will influence future patients' lives. Some occupational therapy faculty prefer to continue to have a clinical practice degree while beginning a career in academia, which is the best of both worlds and keeps them well informed about practice, policy, and changes to health care.

Moving From Practice to Education

Interviewing

The move from clinical practice to academia begins by securing an interview. The first interview is conducted by a search committee composed of members of the hiring department, interdisciplinary faculty, and a student representative. The committee may include the dean but almost always includes the program director.

Preparation

The interview is a give-and-take interchange, as candidates are interviewees and interviewers, and both are interested in determining candidates' fit within the organization. Candidates should prepare by researching the institution's mission, vision, academic programs, accreditation status, faculty credentials, university hierarchy, and cabinet stability. Candidates should ask: Where does the occupational therapy program fit? Is it a school, department, or program within the institution? Who is on the occupational therapy organizational chart? Who are the program's administrators and senior faculty?

Candidates should learn about faculty research to determine similar interests, such as practice areas, graduating institutions, and organization support. These areas can serve as "ice breakers" to begin making connections with faculty.

Thoughtful consideration should be given to any difficulties candidates have encountered as students or obstacles they successfully overcame as practitioners. Conflict is inevitable, and it is important to recognize how one historically handled this as a student and clinician. One primary goal of an interview is to explore interviewees' effectiveness at managing conflict and promoting positive outcomes. The ability to demonstrate serious and creative problem solving, to facilitate change through innovative leadership ideas, and to strengthen relationships among the parties involved are significant areas to explore (Clark et al., 2010; Cranford, 2013).

Candidates must be prepared to talk about their teaching philosophy and with which occupational therapy theories they identify or have used as a framework to advance practice. Interviewees must discuss why they align with a theory and apply it to the faculty position and teaching philosophy. As the interview continues, candidates may be asked about faculty attributes they have admired or disliked while completing graduate school and to discuss these characteristics, identifying those they have or are developing. It is essential to understand that individual qualities can evolve and thus to recognize changes in one's self.

Candidates may be asked about opinions on professional issues related to current research or scholarly interests, work history, including teaching experience, and professional associations and activities. The curriculum vitae should reflect contributions made to the occupational therapy profession, including past mentoring or committee or volunteer work. Diversity in interprofessional contributions or outside the profession is a plus. Candidates should express the value they can add to the institution, which helps them reflect on why they want to work at a specific college or university. It is helpful to write questions that reflect willingness and to have answers ready to respond to the question: Why should we hire you?

Questions to Ask

Candidates should feel comfortable inquiring about what is expected of faculty during the first semester, whether the position is new, and what challenges they might encounter. Candidates should ask about what the committee feels their department does well and what they want to change or improve. Can a syllabus be used as a starting point for the course they will be teaching? If no syllabus is available, how does one access resources to assist with syllabus development? What time is provided for developing or revising the syllabus? What is the approval process? Who makes the final approval about course content?

It is essential that candidates understand the responsibilities of teaching and service. What is the teaching load for this position? Is the position tenured? How are departmental responsibilities, such as committee assignments and advising, divided among faculty? What is considered service, and are faculty provided release time to participate in service?

Candidates also will want to understand the institution's requirements for participation in scholarly activities for tenured and nontenured positions. Is there support for practice-based scholarship? Is there institutional funding to assist in initiating or continuing research? For tenured positions, how are teaching, research, and service ranked in importance for promotion and tenure? What is the average time that faculty spend in each academic rank? How long before assistant professors are reviewed for promotion and tenure?

Toward the end of the interview, candidates should ask about expected salary and benefits to clarify the faculty contract's length, whether it is a 9-, 10-, or 12-month position, and how compensation is paid. Some institutions offer a 10-month faculty contract with a separate opportunity to teach during the summer. Finally, candidates should ask about the committee's expected timeline for making the hiring decision.

Reflection

Once the interview is completed, candidates should reflect on whether they would be happy joining the institution and if they would like to perform the responsibilities discussed. Do they see an opportunity to develop as a scholar? Would experienced faculty provide helpful mentoring? Aligning expectations from the beginning during the interview process will bolster confidence and support satisfaction and long-term success. If significant desired professional benefits are not available, candidates may not find the opportunity to be a good match.

Educational Preparation

Transitioning from clinical practice to academia means making the counterintuitive return to novice from expert. A critical consideration is whether one's degree is an acceptable terminal degree for an institution. Both master's- and doctoral-level occupational therapy graduates are equipped for clinical practice roles; however, they may lack formal education in pedagogy (i.e., teaching methods and practice) or have never reflected on nor developed a teaching philosophy (Table 11-1).

Some doctoral programs (see Table 11-2) may not include courses in pedagogy. Despite the lack of formal training in pedagogy, master's- and doctoral-prepared occupational therapists are actively hired to fill the growing number of vacant academic faculty positions.

The distinctive "language" of education and research sets academia apart from clinical practice. The need for academic integration and socialization will most likely lead to pursuing educational opportunities that differ from previously selected areas of clinical practice. Institutions and programs may have additional educational requirements depending on their needs and candidates' professional experience. Clinicians can further their education with on-campus and online learning courses, conferences, fellowships, certifications, and microbadges.

Traditionally, academic institutions prefer the Doctor of Philosophy (PhD) as the terminal degree for entering academia. Most, if not all, individuals with PhDs are afforded tenured positions, while those with professional doctorate degrees may be offered tenured, nontenured, or clinical lines. The advantage of having a PhD, according to traditional standards for academic rigor, is the ability to disseminate and teach research activities. For example, PhD curricula dedicate more than 50% of their credits toward research learning, while professional doctorates dedicate 30% or fewer credits toward research learning and outcomes (Beres, 2006; McDonald, 2010). PhD students must complete a candidacy exam and dissertation while students seeking professional doctorate degrees complete a scholarly project.

It also is essential to distinguish between the advanced occupational therapy professional doctorate (i.e., post-professional Doctor of Occupational Therapy [PPOTD]) and the first professional doctorate (i.e., entry-level Doctor of Occupational Therapy). Both require completing independent research or scholarly projects. Research projects required to complete an advanced professional doctorate are seldom in an area of discovery but are more so in clinical applications, integration of knowledge, and teaching and learning. Moreover, the first professional doctorate's primary focus is to prepare competent students to enter clinical practice and become eligible for licensure.

Currently, a significant number of PPOTD programs prepare and train qualified occupational therapy clinicians to fill faculty vacancies and increase the number of trained therapists entering academia. PPOTD programs are worth exploring if one is planning to pursue any advanced occupational therapy degree and wants to take education courses.

TABLE 11-1

Common Teaching Methods

METHOD	BRIEF DESCRIPTION	EXAMPLES
Active learning	Course instructor provides structured activities in which students, individually or in groups, engage in tasks related to course content.	Think–Pair–Share Questions embedded into PowerPoint (Microsoft) 1-minute papers Case-based learning
Experiential learning	Course instructor provides authentic, immersive student experiences designed to include reflection.	Field trips Service learning Internships Simulations
Cooperative learning	Course instructor creates small teams of students who work together to accomplish shared group goals and each team member is held responsible and accountable.	Jigsaw Digital collaboration (e.g., Flipgrid [Microsoft], Padlet [Wallwisher, Inc], Diigo [Diigo, Inc])
Inquiry-based instruction	Course instructor encourages and guides students to explore topics and help guide their questions, ideas, and observations. Emphasis is on the student's role in learning.	Problem-based learning Group projects Research projects
Modeling	Course instructor demonstrates a new concept or skill for students, and students observe and then demonstrate.	Demonstration of physical skills Demonstration of patient interview Demonstration of assessment tool
Student-led classroom	Course instructor involves students in planning, implementation, and assessment. The student takes on the role as instructor.	Student presents concepts to classmates using various teaching strategies (e.g., creating lectures, videos, PowerPoint)

Salary and Benefits

Salaries in academia are generally lower than those in clinical practice. This incongruity may be one reason for the dire shortage and older age of occupational therapy faculty. Clinical practice often occurs in a defined time structure and space, but academic requirements can lead to extended work hours and long weeks, including weekends, all on a set salary (Beres, 2006).

TABLE 11-2

PhD Versus Professional Practice Doctorate Degrees

	PHD	ADVANCED PROFESSIONAL DOCTORATE (PPOTD, DNP)	FIRST PROFESSIONAL DOCTORATE (OTD-DPT, PHARMD, MD)	GRADUATE ENTRY-LEVEL PROFESSIONAL DEGREES (PA, MSOT)	CLASSIC MASTER'S DEGREES
> 50% credits are research related[a]	X				
< 30% credits are research related		X	X	X	X
Candidacy exam	X				
Dissertation	X				
Teach and apply evidence-based practice	X	X	X	X	X
Independent research project/outcome[b]	X	X	X	X	X
Translational or implementational research[c]	X	X	X		X
Clinical expertise		X	X	X	
Board certification and licensure to practice—first credential		X	X	X	

[a]Research credits include coursework on research design and statistics and credits assigned to the dissertation, candidacy exam, and doctoral seminar.

[b]For independent research projects/outcomes, students must develop a research question, review the literature, explain the research methodology, collect and interpret the data, and produce a scholarly paper that meets program expectations. The end product may be the scholarly manuscript, a full dissertation, or a sequence of manuscripts based on the collected data. The type of research is comprehensive, including retrospective, outcomes, survey, and future research.

[c]For translational or implementation research, students learn the structure of research design, statistics, and evidence-based practice principles to read research literature and critically apply readings to clinical decision making.

Compensation should be commensurate with experience and workload expectations. For example, an assistant professor in a tenured line and an assistant professor in a nontenured line have different workloads and expectations. Faculty on tenured lines must satisfy teaching, service, and research responsibilities (Clark et al., 2010). Faculty on nontenured lines are responsible mostly for teaching, service, and other departmental activities.

Benefit packages are generally available only for full-time employees. Merit increases, cost-of-living adjustments, and the possibility for promotion should be explored before acceptance. Finally, reimbursement of continuing education, conference attendance, licensure, and certification fees, as well as travel funds, should be determined.

Mentorship

The current exodus in academia has been attributed to the aging of current occupational therapy faculty and inadequate strategic planning to prepare future faculty. Mentorship, one of the most critical roles for department chairs and program directors, can inspire, encourage, support, educate, and promote the necessary growth to sustain novice educators' learning process. Experienced educators can assist with socialization within the institution by providing guidance and insight into department committees' purpose and function. Mentors also can facilitate the process of becoming acquainted with interdisciplinary partnerships and the institutional hierarchy.

Successful mentor–mentee relationships are based on delineating clear goals and expectations for both individuals. Open and honest communication and a commitment of time and energy from both parties is required (Eller et al., 2014; Marfell et al, 2017). Communications should have clear agendas, and meetings should be scheduled regularly.

Conversations should begin with a follow-up from the previous meeting and any issues or ongoing project details. Structured meetings afford the most efficient use of time and provide a historical imprint of knowledge development and growth within the new role. A mentoring journal is a self-reflective tool for preserving all ideas, suggestions, and projects and can help when developing mentees' short- and long-term goals and outcomes.

Facilitating successful mentor–mentee relationships involves essential traits and academic interests. The level of academic knowledge development needs of the mentee and the mentor's academic interests are essential components of the relationship. Scholarly and clinical interests, course assignments, teaching schedules, leadership, learning, and communication styles should be considered when formulating the dyad (Gardner et al., 2019). Some mentors propose that mentees complete an assessment before formalizing a relationship (e.g., StrengthsFinders 2.0, Myers–Briggs Type Indicator, 360 Leadership), which can provide information about how an individual accomplishes goals, learns, leads, and engages in work.

A supportive environment combined with frequent, unbiased feedback encourages mentees in their new role and decreases the levels of anxiety that comes from being a novice. Formal teaching preparation and clear purpose when navigating academic culture can contribute to a successful transition.

New faculty should be allowed to co-teach with experienced faculty before developing and teaching a course alone. The use of well-developed rubrics when grading student work provides an opportunity for the novice to assess students' feedback. At first, novice faculty may find it challenging to deal with a problematic student situation. Having the program director or experienced faculty member review the situation and proposed solutions embedded in academic policies and procedures will provide novices with the skills needed to understand the process and move toward greater academic independence.

Formal seminars to improve teaching skills are essential. Information about the institution's learning management system (e.g., Blackboard [Blackboard, Inc], Canvas [Instructure, Inc], D2L [D2L Incorporation]), library resources, and other tools used to deliver course content and competencies before receiving a student assignment is critical.

Clinical practice has a much different culture than higher education. Academic expectations typically include teaching, scholarship, and service, depending on the academic appointment. Teaching requires syllabus generation, exam construction and analysis, curriculum development, understanding professional standards and guidelines, classroom management, and advising students. Scholarship and service are outlined differently by institution. Mentors can help novice faculty develop a scholarship and service plan and identify sustainable resources.

Institutional Identity

For nearly 5 decades, the Carnegie Classification (Kosar & Scott, 2018) has been the leading framework for recognizing and describing institutional differences in the United States. This framework groups universities according to research, size, and program configuration. Beyond describing institutional differences, this framework also is used to explore research studies' design to ensure adequate representation of sampled institutions, students, or faculty.

Nevertheless, requirements for academic faculty can vary greatly. Candidates should consider overall compatibility (e.g., mission, vision, religious or other institutional affiliations, innovation in program curricula, resources, leadership stability) and explore the program's position within the local community, as well as the school's reputation and ranking.

Team Member Roles and Responsibilities

Joining the academic team may be the most natural part of the passage from the clinic to higher education because occupational therapists have habitual interactions with patients and their family members and other health care providers, which require constant fine-tuning of the delivery of quality patient-centered care. The academic milieu has similar teamwork expectations. Educators are asked to work with a team of faculty to create courses, develop syllabi and competencies, assess students, and undertake other faculty-related tasks identified by the program director, chair, or dean. Cultural differences between practice and education may initially prevent or delay a personal sense of belonging, but it is hoped that any uncertainty in acculturation to the faculty role will be short lived.

Most often, successful teams develop questions to delineate roles and responsibilities when co-teaching. Among these include each faculty member's role in the course, including team leader. What resources are required and available, who will present what content, and in what order will the content be presented? The team also will consider evaluation methods, including how the exam questions are generated and reviewed. Course deployment and all communications must be established and consistently shared with all faculty and students associated with the course, including addressing any technical or delivery problems and student issues.

Teaching and Learning

Education is focused on learner-centered activities. Many definitions of these activities exist; however, at their core are student learning outcomes. Learning in a student-centered environment involves active participation and careful examination of learning outcomes by both faculty and students. Current technology affords much information in this area.

Higher education is in a state of dynamic change, emphasizing how students evaluate and apply content in specific situations, particularly in the health sciences (Barron & Darling-Hammond, 2008). Course competencies within the curriculum are one way that faculty and students can determine learning outcomes and the level of skill acquired.

It is no longer considered good pedagogy to impart passive knowledge in the classroom (American Association of Colleges for Teacher Education, 2008). The knowledge and skills required to apply course content may be taught using a variety of methods, including active, experiential, or cooperative learning; inquiry-based instruction; modeling; and student-led classroom (Barron & Bell, 2015).

Measuring Student Learning

Student success is measured by carefully developed evaluation rubrics that guide student self-assessment and reflection on specific learning outcomes. Through both, students can determine which learning area requires further review or practice to gain the highest level of achievement. Assessments are essential tools to evaluate students' current understanding of knowledge and skills. A variety of structured learning opportunities must be provided to allow students to improve their knowledge of and skills with the established learning outcome.

Assessments must be formative and summative, with assigned grades to be defined and understood metrics. In a study, it was found that in a biology class in which two groups of students were taught the same content, students in a highly structured, student-centered class had significantly higher exam scores and content scores in the post-exam period than did those in a moderately student-centered class (Connell et al., 2016; Stafford-Brizard, 2016). Students from the student-centered group also demonstrated higher expert attitudes toward learning biology as compared to those in the moderately structured class.

Student-centered learning aims to explore what students have learned. Analysis of content and learning success includes whether the established learning outcomes were met and the achievement level. This shift in pedagogy is from emphasizing what students are taught instead of what they learn during their educational journey (Osher et al., 2018; Stafford-Brizard, 2016).

Developing Curricula

The same way occupational therapists collaborate with other health care practitioners to assess, treat, and manage clients' rehabilitation, occupational therapy faculty work with other team members to develop curricula that reflect best practices in how therapists are educated. Such work is rarely done in isolation. For occupational therapy–centered courses, faculty typically work in curriculum committees with their colleagues. These committees review current best practices in both disciplines and approaches to teaching, emphasizing how the curriculum supports the mission and goals of the program, department, school, and university, as well as the profession.

Faculty regularly consult national practice standards. For example, occupational therapy curricula are informed by the American Occupational Therapy Association (AOTA), which provides information on current health care policies, reimbursement, and best practices; the Accreditation Council for Occupational Therapy Education (2018), which publishes the essential accreditation standards for all occupational therapy programs; and by the National Board for Certification in Occupational Therapy, which provides the certification exam required for new graduates to practice occupational therapy. Together, these entities delineate the knowledge and skills or practice competencies for occupational therapy entry. Their documents also are used to evaluate occupational therapy programs for accreditation.

Occupational therapy faculty may engage in interprofessional educational initiatives, including research and other scholarly activities (Stafford-Bizard et al., 2016), with physical therapy, speech-language pathology, nursing, public health, pharmacy, social work, education and business faculty, physician assistant, and policy experts among a few. Occupational therapists co-teach interprofessional courses with those from other disciplines in some academic settings, including those on anatomy, research, cultural awareness, bioethics, and community practice. Opportunities to collaborate with educators from other professions can be rewarding, particularly for those therapists who like to address matters from a broad perspective (McDonald, 2010).

Accreditation

Accreditation is the primary way higher education institutions "assure and improve the quality of higher education institutions" (Higher Leaning Commission, n.d.; Kajaste et al., 2015). In the United States, most colleges and universities seek accreditation by a regional accreditor approved by

TABLE 11-3

U.S. Institutional Accrediting Agencies

ACCREDITING AGENCY	PRIMARY REGIONS OR STATES SERVED
Accrediting Commission for Community and Junior Colleges (2020)	California, Hawaii, and the Pacific Region (Guam, American Samoa, the Republic of Palau, the Federated States of Micronesia, the Republic of the Marshall Islands, and the Commonwealth of the Northern Marianas Islands)
Higher Learning Commission (n.d.)	Arizona, Arkansas. Colorado, Illinois, Indiana, Iowa, Kansas, Michigan, Minnesota, Missouri, Nebraska, New Mexico, North Dakota, Ohio, Oklahoma, South Dakota, West Virginia, Wisconsin, and Wyoming
Middle States Commission on Higher Education (2022)	Delaware, the District of Columbia, Maryland, New Jersey, New York, Pennsylvania, Puerto Rico, and the U.S. Virgin Islands Includes distance education and correspondence education programs offered at those institutions
New England Association of Schools and Colleges (2020)	Connecticut, Maine, Massachusetts, New Hampshire, Rhode Island, and Vermont
Southern Association of Colleges and Schools Commission on Colleges (2020)	Alabama, Florida, Georgia, Kentucky, Louisiana, Mississippi, North Carolina, South Carolina, Tennessee, Texas, Virginia, and Latin America and other international sites approved by the commission that award associate, baccalaureate, master's, or doctoral degrees
Northwest Commission on Colleges and Universities (2020)	Alaska, Idaho, Montana, Nevada, Oregon, Utah, and Washington
Western Association of Schools and Colleges Senior College and University Commission (2020)	California, Hawaii, and the Pacific Region, as well as a limited number of institutions outside the United States

the Department of Education. Seven active accreditation agencies in the United States have received such recognition (Table 11-3).

Just as colleges and universities seek accreditation to ensure the ongoing quality of their offerings, occupational therapy programs seek accreditation to confirm that these programs meet rigorous standards that support the profession and improve patient outcomes. In addition, many state occupational therapy licensure agencies and several graduate programs mandate that an applicant for licensure or admission into a program must have graduated from an accredited occupational therapy occupational therapy program.

Most state occupational therapy licensure boards require initial program approval to ensure that occupational therapy students meet all established education requirements. Universities, colleges, and occupational therapy programs receive an initial accreditation status and are reviewed on a schedule to ensure the maintenance of quality education standards. These formal reviews require a written report and a site visit performed by representatives of the accrediting agency.

Currently, the Department of Education recognizes the Accreditation Council for Occupational Therapy Education as the occupational therapy accrediting body for all entry-level occupational therapy education: associate, baccalaureate, master's, and entry-level doctoral programs.

An Urgent Need

Faculty positions in occupational therapy are increasingly challenging to fill and growing unfilled each year. The academic shortage can be traced to several causes, including a lack of mentorship for candidates entering higher education and perceived lower salaries compared to responsibilities.

In 2015, AOTA conducted a salary workforce survey providing detailed information across practice areas. Among the areas surveyed were preferred practice settings; only 0.3% of occupational therapists selected academia as their first choice for practice. In 2019, AOTA again conducted a second salary workforce survey method asking for anticipating shortage or surplus of faculty, and 88.1% (of 126) of the responders selected anticipating a future shortage of faculty. These responses are primarily due to a limited pool of doctorally prepared faculty and a lack of faculty with the right specialty mix to fit diverse occupational therapy programs' needs. Additional factors identified in these surveys include the aging of current faculty, a wave of anticipated faculty retirements in the next 10 years, and higher compensation in the clinical and private sectors (AOTA, 2010, 2015, 2019). Even with doctoral degrees, lower wages and family obligations can lead many clinicians to transition to academia much later in their careers.

References

Accreditation Council for Occupational Therapy Education. (2018). Accreditation Council for Occupational Therapy Education (ACOTE) standards and interpretive guide (effective July 31, 2020). *American Journal of Occupational Therapy, 72*(Suppl. 2), 7212410005p1–7212410005p83. https://doi.org/10.5014/ajot.2018.72S217

Accrediting Commission for Community and Junior Colleges. (2020). *About us.* http://accjc.org/about/

American Association of Colleges for Teacher Education. (2008). *Handbook of technological pedagogical content knowledge (TPCK) for educators.* Routledge.

American Occupational Therapy Association. (2010). *Faculty workforce survey* [PDF]. AOTA Press. https://www.aota.org/~/media/Corporate/Files/EducationCareers/Educators/OTEdData/2010%20Faculty%20Survey%20Report.pdf

American Occupational Therapy Association. (2015). *Salary workforce survey.* AOTA Press.

American Occupational Therapy Association. (2019). *2019 salary workforce survey methods.* AOTA Press.

Barron, B., & Bell, P. (2015). Learning environments in and out of school. In D. C. Berliner & R. C. Calfee (Eds.), *Handbook of educational psychology* (pp. 323–336). Routledge.

Barron, B., & Darling-Hammond, L. (2008). How can we teach for meaningful learning? In L. Darling-Hammond, *Powerful learning: What we know about teaching for understanding.* Jossey-Bass.

Beres, J. (2006). Staff development to university faculty: Reflections of a nurse educator. *Nursing Forum, 41*(3), 141-145. https://doi.org/10.1111/j.1744-6198.2006.00050.x

Clark, N. J., Alcala-Van Houten, L., & Perea-Ryan, M. (2010). Transitioning from clinical practice to academia: University expectations on the tenure track. *Nurse Educator, 35*(3), 105-109. https://doi.org/10.1097/NNE.0b013e3181d95069

Connell, G. L., Donovan, D. A., & Chambers, T. G. (2016). Increasing the use of student-centered pedagogies from moderate to high improves student learning and attitudes about biology. *CBE—Life Sciences Education, 15*(1). https://doi.org/10.1187/cbe.15-03-0062

Cranford, J. S. (2013). Bridging the gap: Clinical practice nursing and the effect of role strain on successful role transition and intent to stay in academia. *International Journal of Nursing Education Scholarship, 10,* 99–105. https://doi.org/10.1515/ijnes-2012-0018

Eller, L. A., Lev, E. L., & Feurer, A. (2014). Key components of an effective mentoring relationship: A qualitative study. *Nurse Education Today, 34*(5), 815-820. https://doi.org/10.1016/j.nedt.2013.07.020

Gardner, A. L., Clementz, L., Lawrence, R. H., Dolansky, M. A., Heilman, A. M., Rusterholtz, A. R., Singh, S., Sparks, M., & Singh, M. K. (2019). The dyad model for interprofessional academic patient aligned care teams. *Federal Practitioner: For the Health Care Professionals of the VA, DoD, and PHS, 36*(2), 88–93.

Higher Learning Commission. (n.d.). *About the higher learning commission.* https://www.hlcommission.org/About-the-Commission/about-hlc.html

Kajaste, M., Prades, A., & Scheuthle, H. (2015). Impact evaluation from quality assurance agencies' perspectives: Methodological approaches, experiences and expectations. *Quality in Higher Education, 21*(3), 270-287. https://doi.org/10.1080/13538322.2015.1111006

Kosar, R., & Scott, D. W. (2018). Examining the Carnegie Classification Methodology for research universities. *Statistics and Public Policy, 5*(1), 1-12. https://doi.org/10.1080/2330443X.2018.1442271

Marfell, J., Mc Mullen, P. C., Onieal, M. E., Scheibmeir, M., & Hawkins-Walsh, E. (2017). Key considerations for moving to a nurse faculty role: A dean's perspective. *Journal of the American Association of Nurse Practitioners, 29*(8), 475–483. https://doi.org/10.1002/2327-6924.12489

McDonald, P. J. (2010). Transitioning from clinical practice to nursing faculty: Lessons learned. *Journal of Nursing Education, 49*(3), 126-131. https://doi.org/10.3928/01484834-20091022-02

Middle States Commission on Higher Education. (2022). *About us.* https://www.msche.org

New England Association of Schools and Colleges. (2020). *About NECHE.* https://cihe.neasc.org/

Northwest Commission on Colleges and Universities. (2020). *About NWCCU.* https://nwccu.org/about-nwccu/

Osher, D., Cantor, P., Berg, J., Steyer, L., & Rose, T. (2018). Drivers of human development: How relationships and context shape learning and development. *Applied Developmental Science, 1,* 6-36. https://doi.org/10.1080/10888691.2017.1398650

Southern Association of Colleges and Schools Commission on Colleges. (2020). *About SASCOC.* https://sacscoc.org/about-sacscoc/

Stafford-Brizard, K. (2016). *Nonacademic skills are the necessary foundation for learning.* Education Week. https://www.edweek.org/leadership/opinion-nonacademic-skills-are-the-necessary-foundation-for-learning/2016/07

Vassantachart, D. S. M., & Rice, G. T. (1997). Academic integration of occupational therapy faculty. *American Journal of Occupational Therapy, 51,* 584-588. https://doi.org/10.5014/AJOT.51.7.584

Western Association of Schools and Senior College and University Commission. (2020). *About.* https://www.wscuc.org/about/

Section II

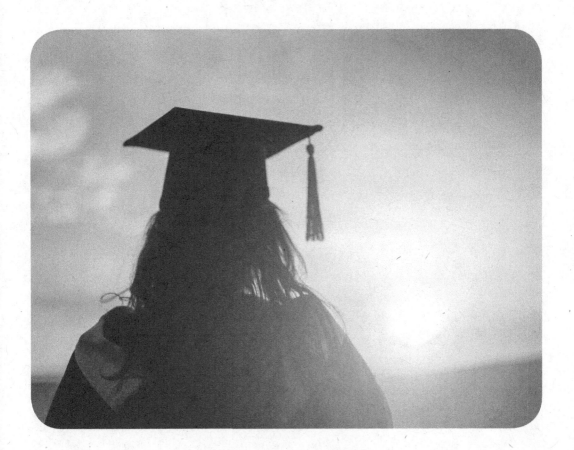

EMERGING
PRACTICE AREAS

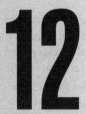

Primary Care

Robin Akselrud, OTD, OTR/L;
Teresa (Tee) Stock, OTD, MSOT, MBA, OTR/L;
and Miriam Wachspress, MS, OTR/L

Primary Care in a Nutshell

Occupational therapy's fit within a primary care setting is a good one, as both view patients in a holistic manner and also focus on promoting a healthy lifestyle and preventing illness and injury. Research and my own personal experiences within a primary care setting, however, indicate a more uneasy fit with specific challenges (R.A.).

Occupational Therapy's Role

Occupational therapists in a primary care setting can collaborate with physicians about patients' individual needs and abilities. Therapists are well trained to treat many diagnoses; therefore, they can be great assets in a primary care setting, providing direct care or consultation with physicians and other health care professionals. Occupational therapists can work with geriatric, pediatric, and adult patient populations.

According to Donnelly et al. (2017, p. 2), "A national survey of occupational therapists working on primary care teams found that the most frequent services being provided were health promotion and prevention activities (71%), including falls prevention (71%) and home safety assessment (69%)." However, occupational therapy has encountered some challenges in primary care. Donnelly et al. (2013) have discussed why the profession often is not integrated into this type of setting. First is a lack of reimbursement for occupational therapy services in this area. Second, occupational therapists most often work as solo practitioners, focusing heavily on the biomechanical or

Akselrud, R. (Ed.). *Quintessential Occupational Therapy:*
A Guide to Areas of Practice (pp 137-144).
© 2023 Taylor & Francis Group.

the rehabilitation model. Third is the lack of physician and staff education about the value of occupational therapy and how therapists collaborate in patient overall health and well-being. With an increased emphasis on interprofessional primary care, professions such as occupational therapy should be integrated into more primary health care settings to benefit patients.

Patient skills addressed in occupational therapy interventions are individualized. For example, children may be treated for areas of deficit, such as low muscle tone, developmental delays, poor handwriting skills, and posture issues. Adults may be treated for injuries of the hand, chronic pain, or mental illness. Senior patients may need training in cognition, activities of daily living (ADLs), and transfers.

Evaluation

Occupational therapy practitioners can be involved in evaluations in the primary care setting through consults, screenings, and full evaluations. They often assist in or carry out the initial intakes. The occupational therapy practitioner could begin with an initial intake form such as that shown in Figure 12-1 or by using an occupational profile template (American Occupational Therapy Association [AOTA], 2020) and/or the Canadian Occupational Performance Measure (Donnelly et al., 2017). Examples of a primary care occupational therapy screen and occupational therapy evaluation form for a child are shown in Figures 12-2 and 12-3, respectively.

Intervention

Based upon the occupational needs and goals of the client found during the evaluation, the occupational therapist would plan interventions as part of a collaborative team. Interventions might include patient and/or family education, medication management, discussing implications of chronic illness, working on functional cognition, addressing safety, prevention of rehospitalizations, management of musculoskeletal conditions, and increasing independence in daily activities (AOTA, 2020). According to AOTA (2020, p. 3), "Occupational therapy practitioners make a distinct contribution in primary care by recognizing and addressing the impact of roles, habits, and routines on management of chronic conditions and development of healthy lifestyles. Occupational therapy practitioners also play a significant role in lifestyle modification for chronic disease management." Occupational therapy practitioners can also play a key role in addressing mental and behavioral health as it relates to client occupations (AOTA, 2020).

Discharge Planning or Transitioning

Occupational therapists involved in primary care can help ensure clients are safe to be discharged, have accommodations and adaptive equipment in place, and have access to community resources and support. The occupational therapist can help make community referrals to provide continuity of care (AOTA, 2020).

Tips and Advice From the Field

Occupational therapists planning to work in primary care settings should understand care delivery and payment models that may apply in this setting. According to AOTA (2020, p. 7), "..two main categories of reimbursement in primary care exist: (1) relative value unit, or fee-for-service, and (2) value-based payment." To successfully engage in primary care, occupational therapy practitioners must be aware of the payment models within their setting and ensure that the delivery model for occupational therapy services is reimbursable. Many challenges come with advocating for reimbursement, including payment criteria and regulations. Being prepared to address reimbursement and regulatory issues, however, is part of the current role of occupational therapy practitioners entering primary care. We are well-suited as practitioners in this area of practice due to our holistic

Patient name:
Date of birth:
Medical diagnosis:

General Medical Information
Have you had any surgeries?
Do you experience any pain in your hands? Neck? Back?
How is your posture?
Do you experience any tingling or numbness in your hands? Wrists? Shoulders?
Do you have any trouble with balance? Any history of falls?

ADLs and IADLs
Can you dress and undress yourself without help from others?
Can you dress and bathe/take a bath or shower without help from others?
Can you get in and out of bed without help from others?
Can you cook/clean/shop by yourself without help from others?
Do you have any difficulty opening and closing buttons and zippers?
Do you have difficulty opening containers or jars?
Do you have difficulty with writing?
Do your hands get tired quickly from writing or from using them for daily activities?
Are there any activities or daily tasks that you would like to perform better? Are there any that you cannot complete yourself?

Cognition and Mental Health
Do you have trouble with memory? Do you forget often?
Do you have feelings of depression or anxiety?
Do you have difficulty in social situations? Maintaining eye contact and conversation?
Are you easily distracted?

Figure 12-1. Sample occupational therapy primary care screening for adolescents and adults.

approach and our educational background, which covers social, mental, physical, biological, and behavioral sciences (AOTA, 2020). Occupational therapists should be prepared to explain their value to the patient and primary care team.

The AOTA offers many recent documents and resources for this emerging niche. Among these resources is the AOTA *Position Statement on the Role of Occupational Therapy in Primary Care* (AOTA, 2020). Other helpful articles and resources include:

- *Practice Settings: Primary Care*: https://www.aota.org/practice/practice-settings/primary-care (AOTA, 2022)
- *Providing Occupational Therapy in a Free Primary Care Clinic*: https://www.aota.org/publications/ot-practice/ot-practice-issues/2019/free-primary-clinic (White et al., 2019)
- *Canadian Occupational Performance Measure in Primary Care: A Profile of Practice* (Donnelly et al., 2017)
- *Role of Occupational Therapy in Pediatric Primary Care: Promoting Childhood Development* (Riley et al., 2021)

Child's name: _____

Child's age: _____

The following questions are posed to help our team of professionals obtain a complete picture of your child from early infancy to their present developmental stage. Some questions may refer to children who are older than your own. Check the choice that applies: Yes or No. Please add any important narrative information in the comments section.

Any complications with pregnancy? _____

If premature, how early? _____

	Yes	No	Comments
Was the child born through Cesarean section?			
Was the child born breech (feet first)?			
Was the umbilical cord wrapped around the child's neck?			
Were forceps required?			
Did the child have feeding problems as a newborn?			

Were feeding and sleeping patterns easily established? Yes or No. If not, please explain.

_____

When did your child consistently sleep through the night?

_____

Fussy baby past 6 months of age? Yes or No. If yes, any reason identified?

_____

Indicate the child's age for achieving the skill. If uncertain, indicate early, late, or typical:

_____ Independent sitting   _____ Hands/knees crawling   _____ Walking

_____ First words   _____ Sentences   _____ Toilet trained

Do you think that any part of your child's development is slower than average? If yes, please explain.

_____

Check the following items that best describe your child:

Visual Skills

_____ Wears glasses

_____ Has been diagnosed with a visual problem (describe):

_____ Has difficulty finding/seeing things (e.g., shoes in the closet, toy in a toy basket)

Figure 12-2. Sample primary care occupational therapy pediatric screening. *(continued)*

Auditory and Language Skills

_____ Has a suspected/diagnosed hearing loss
_____ Limited or absence of gesturing to assist communication
_____ Excessive talking interferes with listening
_____ Nonverbal

Oral–Motor and Respiratory Control

_____ Displays poor lip control for eating, using utensils
_____ Chokes easily on liquids or solids
_____ Has limited skills with blow toys, bubbles
_____ Overstuffs mouth with food
_____ Demonstrates poor saliva control (drools)
_____ Clenches jaw or grinds teeth

Self-Care/Regulation of Body Function

Is your child able to complete these tasks independently (please circle Yes/No)?

Yes	No	Toileting: bowel/bladder control
Yes	No	Zippers pull/engage/disengage
Yes	No	Velcro on/off
Yes	No	Undresses
Yes	No	Socks on/off
Yes	No	Dresses
Yes	No	Snaps/unsnaps
Yes	No	Buttons
Yes	No	Self-feeding (finger foods)
Yes	No	Uses eating utensils
Yes	No	Uses open cup
Yes	No	Uses a straw
Yes	No	Sippy cup

Sensory Concerns

_____ Becomes fearful, anxious, or aggressive with light or unexpected touch
_____ Complains about having hair brushed, may be picky about using a particular brush
_____ Avoids touching certain textures of material (e.g., blankets, rugs, stuffed animal)
_____ Refuses to wear new, stiff, or rough textured clothes (e.g., turtlenecks, jeans, hats, belts)
_____ Avoids/dislikes/aversive to "messy play" (e.g., sand, mud, water, glue, glitter, PlayDoh, slime, shaving cream)
_____ May walk only on toes
_____ May crave touch, needing to touch everything and everyone
_____ May be unaware that hands or face are dirty or cannot feel nose running
_____ Mouths objects excessively
_____ May be a messy dresser (e.g., looks disheveled, does not notice pants are twisted, shirt is half untucked, shoes are untied, one pant leg is up and one is down)
_____ Has difficulty using scissors, crayons, or silverware
_____ Avoids/dislikes playground equipment (e.g., swings, ladders, slides, merry-go-rounds)
_____ Afraid of heights, even the height of a curb or step
_____ Loses balance easily and may appear clumsy
_____ In constant motion and cannot seem to sit still

Figure 12-2 (continued). Sample primary care occupational therapy pediatric screening. (continued)

_____ Is a "thrill-seeker," is dangerous at times

_____ Frequently slumps, lies down, or leans head on hand or arm while working at their desk

_____ Fatigues easily

_____ Has poor body awareness (e.g., bumps into things, knocks things over, trips, appears clumsy)

_____ Has difficulty learning exercise or dance steps

_____ Bites or sucks on fingers or frequently cracks knuckles

_____ Chews on pens, straws, or shirt sleeves

_____ Distracted by sounds not normally noticed by others (e.g., humming of lights or refrigerators, fans, heaters, clocks ticking)

_____ Dislikes loud sounds (e.g., vacuum cleaner, toilet flushing, alarms)

_____ Is picky eater, often with extreme food preferences (e.g., limited repertoire of foods, picky about brands, resistive to trying new foods or restaurants, may not eat at other people's houses)

_____ Has difficulty keeping eyes focused on task/activity for an appropriate amount of time

_____ Avoids eye contact

_____ Often loses place when copying from a book or chalkboard

_____ Has difficulty with consistent letter spacing and sizing during writing or lining up numbers in math problems

_____ Has difficulty with jigsaw puzzles, copying shapes, or cutting/tracing along a line

_____ Confuses left and right

Social Skills

_____ Has difficulty getting along with peers

_____ Prefers playing by self with objects or toys rather than with people

_____ Others have a hard time interpreting the child's cues, needs, or emotions

_____ Emotional skills

_____ Has difficulty accepting changes in routine (even having tantrums)

_____ Gets easily frustrated

_____ Is often impulsive

_____ Shows excessive irritability, fussiness, or colic as an infant

_____ Cannot calm or soothe self through pacifier, comfort object, or caregiver

_____ Requires excessive help from caregiver to fall asleep (e.g., rubbing back or head, rocking, long walks, car rides)

Figure 12-2 (continued). Sample primary care occupational therapy pediatric screening.

Schedule and Caseload

The daily schedule in a primary care setting can vary, but most operate from early morning to early evening during the week. Many facilities allow for walk-in visits, but others may require an appointment in advance. Because specialists and other health care providers often work in the same facility, presenting diagnoses typically vary as well. A typical caseload includes patients of all ages.

Child's name: _____

Date of birth: _____

Diagnosis:

Medical history:

Birth history:

Developmental history/milestones:

Peabody Developmental Motor Scales score: _____

Lifting head: _____

Rolling over: _____

Sitting: _____

Crawling: _____

Walking: _____

Muscle tone: _____

Muscle strength: _____

Posture: _____

Prewriting/writing skills: _____

Grasping skills/grasp pattern/hand dominance: _____

Scissor skills: _____

Visual Motor Integration score: _____

Visual–perceptual skills: _____

Visual–motor skills: _____

Tracking: _____

Scanning: _____

Figure–ground discrimination: _____

Depth perception: _____

Form constancy: _____

Visual memory: _____

Visual closure: _____

Motor control/praxis: _____

Sensory integration deficits: _____

Sensory Profile score: _____

Hypersensitivity/hyposensitivity: _____

ADLs skills: _____

Attention/focus to task: _____

Eye contact: _____

Parent/teacher concerns:

Recommendations:

Figure 12-3. Sample occupational therapy primary care evaluation for children.

Suitability for Practice

The fast-paced primary care setting may be suitable for new graduates only if supervision is readily available. Students or practitioners changing fields can try to seek out new placements in this niche area of practice with the guidance of university staff or experienced practitioners. They can seek a mentor who is practicing in this setting through their state organization or through AOTA CommunOT (https://communot.aota.org/home). Occupational therapists working in primary care must be flexible to changes in caseload and schedule and must be comfortable with educating other medical professionals and staff about the profession and its roles.

References

American Occupational Therapy Association. (2020). Role of occupational therapy in primary care. *American Journal of Occupational Therapy, 74*(Suppl. 3), 7413410040p1–7413410040p16. https://doi.org/10.5014/ajot.2020.74S3001

American Occupational Therapy Association. (2022). *Practice settings: Primary care.* https://www.aota.org/practice/practice-settings/primary-care

Donnelly, C., Brenchley, C., Crawford, C., & Letts, L. (2013). The integration of occupational therapy into primary care: A multiple case study design. *BMC Family Practice, 14,* 60. https://doi.org/10.1186/1471-2296-14-60

Donnelly, C., O'Neill, C., Bauer, M., & Letts, L. (2017). Canadian Occupational Performance Measure (COPM) in primary care: A profile of practice. *American Journal of Occupational Therapy, 71*(6), 7106265010p1-7106265010p8. https://doi.org/10.5014/ajot.2017.020008

Riley, B. R. W., & de Sam Lazaro, S. L. (2021). Role of occupational therapy in pediatric primary care: Promoting childhood development. *American Journal of Occupational Therapy, 75*(6), 7506090010. https://doi.org/10.5014/ajot.2021.756002

White, J., Toto, P., Skidmore, E., & Baker, N. (2019). *Providing occupational therapy in a free primary care clinic.* AOTA. https://www.aota.org/publications/ot-practice/ot-practice-issues/2019/free-primary-clinic

13

Community Settings

Lee Westover, MS, OTR/L

Community Settings in a Nutshell

Occupational therapy originated in mental health treatment settings. Although for many years occupational therapy's presence in this practice area has been decreasing, it is again growing and has never been more essential.

During the 1960s civil rights movement, large psychiatric hospitals began to implement policies that were meant to integrate people with mental illness or other disabilities into the community and out of long-term institutional care (Yohanna et al., 2013). Although this movement, known as *deinstitutionalization*, was well-intended, a lack of affordable housing and treatment options for people with severe mental illness resulted in an increasing number of individuals with severe needs being "housed" in prisons and homeless shelters (Aurand et al., 2020). Occupational therapists in community settings (e.g., shelters, substance use treatment, supportive housing, primary care clinics, prisons) are beginning to utilize the profession's unique support of individuals' ability to function and fulfill life roles in the community across the lifespan.

Approximately 568,000 people experienced homelessness in the United States on any given night in 2019 (U.S. Department of Housing and Urban Development, 2020). Individuals experiencing homelessness endure much higher rates of disability and mental illness, earlier death, and less access to supportive services than does the general population (Dams-O'Conner et al., 2014).

Akselrud, R. (Ed.). *Quintessential Occupational Therapy:
A Guide to Areas of Practice* (pp 145-156).
© 2023 Taylor & Francis Group.

Cognitive impairment is frequently present and is a hallmark symptom of traumatic brain injury (Centers for Disease Control and Prevention, 2019; Stubbs et al., 2020). More than 53% of people who are homeless have experienced a traumatic brain injury during their lifetime, almost half of those injuries were moderate to severe, and up to 92% of people sustained the injury before becoming homeless (Stubbs et al., 2020). These rates are even higher for veterans (Barnes et al., 2015; U.S. Interagency Council on Homelessness, 2018) and individuals who have been incarcerated (U.S. Department of Health and Human Services Centers for Disease Control and Prevention, 2007).

Histories of trauma interlaced with substance use disorder and societal stigma underlie complex interactions of ability and disability. Many individuals move among prisons, shelters, outpatient and inpatient mental health settings, and housing programs for years. Occupational therapists in community settings work with people who experience these qualities at any given time, so therapeutic use of self for rapport building, functional and cognitive assessment, skills development training, environmental adaptation expertise, and application of health care and housing policy can make for a rich and holistic occupational therapy practice.

Occupational Therapy's Role

Recommendations for occupational therapy practice in Chapter 8 of this book can also be applied to a career in a community setting. However, specific areas of knowledge should be utilized to support patients with histories of substance use disorder, incarceration, and homelessness in achieving their optimal level of independence in the community.

Recovery

As with mental health settings in general, a recovery orientation is also essential in community settings. According to the Substance Abuse and Mental Health Services Administration's (2012) definition, *recovery* is "a process of change through which individuals improve their health and wellness, live a self-directed life, and strive to reach their full potential" (p. 3). As such, patient-driven community integration should be the focus of practice as it is supportive of long-term maintenance of housing and employment. These goals are often shared by both patients and human services professionals.

Community Integration

Wong and Solomon's (2002) definition of *community integration* includes three overarching domains: physical, social, and psychological integration. *Physical integration* refers to how well people can utilize resources and participate in meaningful activities in the community. *Social integration* includes the *interactional dimension* (ability to engage in culturally normative, everyday social interaction) and *social network dimension* (size and quality of a positive, reciprocal social support network and fulfillment of roles therein). *Psychological integration* represents the degree to which people feel that they belong, can fulfill personal needs, and are emotionally connected to their community. Institutionalization in shelters and prisons, as well as social exclusion resulting from societal stigma, can negatively affect these domains.

A natural first step for occupational therapists in this setting is to first develop strong rapport with patients and then help them identify personal goals. Establishment of rapport may take much time as many of these individuals have learned to distrust human services professionals and others who may have power over them. Goal achievement is supported by maintaining a focus on supporting all domains of community integration and an internal locus of control through all resulting interventions. Progressive practice frameworks, such as the examples that follow, can be applied by therapists to ensure this focus.

Harm Reduction

Principles of harm reduction were initially developed as practical strategies and ideas that are intended to reduce the negative consequences resulting from substance use (Hawk et al., 2017). The main assumptions underlying harm reduction are that individuals who use drugs or participate in other risky behaviors are worthy of respect, self-determination, and protection from harm. Harm reduction supports the idea that risky behaviors are a permanent part of our world, and people engage in these activities for many reasons, including cultural attitudes and environments.

Six main principles were identified in a systematic review by Hawk et al. (2017) as making up the core of the harm reduction framework across health care settings: humanism, pragmatism, individualism, autonomy, incrementalism, and accountability without termination (Table 13-1). The essential values at the core of harm reduction are that people who engage in risky behaviors deserve respect, compassion, and dignity; that they should be meaningfully included in program design and have easy access to the services they desire and require; and that service providers must meet patients "where they are," without judgment, stigma, or coercion. Harm reduction has also been applied to sex work, eating disorders, and tobacco use.

Housing First

Housing First also supports the prioritization of a personalized practice and patient self-determination (U.S. Department of Housing and Urban Development, n.d.). As more people are being housed in institutional settings, the negative effects of acclimation to those settings (e.g., learned helplessness) is becoming better understood. In response, nonprofit housing organizations are utilizing federal funding to support Housing First programs.

A linear approach to housing requires that patients "graduate" from treatment or training programs before they move into housing. Strong research has demonstrated that moving people into housing and *then* providing wraparound supports, often including occupational therapy, increases maintenance of long-term housing and reduces court involvement, emergency department visits, 911 calls, and hospitalizations. Whereas Housing First is backed by evidence as being effective (Goering et al., 2014), it is not yet a default solution to homelessness.

Even so, the guiding principles of the framework can be applied in many settings to emphasize the individualized treatment and support that ensure long-term success for individuals who are homeless. Principles of Housing First can be found in Table 13-2. Patients' needs and desires are prioritized over societal or programmatic priorities. Patients are to be met "where they are," not where providers would like them to be. All individuals deserve respect and a safe place to live, and a home is not something to be earned.

Intersectionality

People of color, LGBTQIA+ individuals, people with disabilities, and indigenous people are all overrepresented in the population of those who experience homelessness. Often, a person who is homeless experiences several of those qualities, resulting in discrimination and stigma from many directions and deep degrees of inequities.

For example, during her life, a woman of color who lives with histories of trauma, mental illness, and poverty may experience discrimination based on stigma regarding her economic, gender, race, disability, and class background. The intersection of these types of discrimination can result in deep and challenging barriers to exiting homelessness. Occupational therapists working with such individuals will need to consider all of these barriers to provide effective services (Marshall et al., 2020).

TABLE 13-1

Principles of Harm Reduction

PRINCIPLE	DEFINITION	APPLICATION
Humanism	Providers respect patients as individuals and treat them as such. They participate in risky behaviors for a reason that must be understood to empower both provider and patient.	Providers do not make moral judgments against patients. Services are responsive to patients' needs and easy to access. Patients' choices are respected, not just tolerated.
Pragmatism	No one achieves perfection. Social and community norms affect how people behave and their ability to change.	Abstinence is not always desired or possible, so a range of approaches should be provided. Protecting from actual harm is more important than meeting societal standards.
Individualism	Everyone presents with a spectrum of their own strengths, deficits, and needs. As such, a spectrum of intervention options should be available to them.	Strengths and needs are individually assessed and assumptions about them should not be made by providers. Communication with patients should be as personally tailored as is the intervention.
Autonomy	Through education about their treatment options, patients can make their own choices about interventions and personal goals.	The relationship between provider and patient should be driven by the patient's priorities and decisions. Both learn from each other in a reciprocal manner.
Incrementalism	Any change toward improved health and well-being is positive, no matter how small. Backward movement away from goal achievement is normal and can be planned for.	Providers help patients celebrate all of their successes, no matter how small, and help them recognize that plateaus and backsliding happen to everyone. Positive reinforcement is essential.
Accountability without termination	Patients, not providers, are responsible for their own lives and choices. Patients are not "fired" for not making progress and have the absolute right to make decisions that are harmful to themselves. Providers can help them understand the consequences of such without judgment.	Punishment for not making progress or backsliding is not acceptable. Providers assist patients in accepting their own progress in their personal contexts.

TABLE 13-2

Principles of Housing First

- Homelessness is first and foremost a housing crisis and can be addressed through the provision of safe, affordable housing.
- All people experiencing homelessness, regardless of their housing history and duration of homelessness, can achieve housing stability in permanent housing. Some may need little support for a brief period while others may need more intensive, longer term supports.
- Everyone is "housing ready." Sobriety, treatment compliance, or even a lack of criminal history is not necessary to succeed in housing. Rather, homelessness programs and housing providers must be "consumer ready."
- Many people experience improvements in quality of life, in the areas of health, mental health, substance use, and employment, as a result of achieving housing.
- People experiencing homelessness have the right to self-determination and should be treated with dignity and respect.
- The exact configuration of housing and services depends on a population's needs and preferences.

Evaluation and Assessments

Canadian Occupational Performance Measure

The Canadian Occupational Performance Measure (COPM) is a flexible, semi-structured interview that explores occupational performance strengths and deficits (Law et al., 2014). Up to five occupational problems are identified by importance and are rated from 1 to 10 for current performance and satisfaction with performance, with 1 = *poor* and 10 = *excellent*.

These problem areas are then converted into personal goals in treatment plans. Every 3 to 6 months, goals are reassessed to determine patient progress. A change score is generated after reassessment, which records progress quantitatively. Any change of two points in either direction is considered significant. The process of exploring a patient's current daily life in such detail can be difficult for some, but if trust has been established, the COPM can contribute significantly to therapeutic rapport by aligning the interests of patient and provider.

Goal Attainment Scaling

Goal Attainment Scaling is a flexible method of allowing patients to track their own progress toward personal goals (Doig et al., 2010). The COPM has been used to identify long-term goals to track using Goal Attainment Scaling. Patients select a goal and work with occupational therapists to determine realistic and achievable steps to take toward attainment. The goal is then scaled up when patients are able to accomplish more than initially thought and down if they fall short of the initial goal. Patients score their own progress and then problem solve (with assistance, if necessary) to create a new set of outcomes (see Table 13-3 for examples). Patients' scoring their own progress supports an internal locus of control for achieving goals.

TABLE 13-3

Goal Attainment Scaling

Long-term goal: Incorporate mindfulness activities into my daily routine.

GOAL ATTAINMENT LEVELS	GOAL BEHAVIOR
Much-more-than-expected outcome (+2).	Participate in a mindfulness activity more than once before the end of the week.
More-than-expected outcome (+1).	Participate in a mindfulness activity before the end of the week.
Expected outcome (0).	Identify two to three mindfulness activities to try this week.
Less-than-expected outcome (−1).	Identify one mindfulness activity to try this week.
Much-less-than-expected outcome (−2).	Research mindfulness activities.

Executive Function Performance Test

The Executive Function Performance Test utilizes observation of four naturalistic activities of daily living or instrumental activities of daily living to evaluate executive function (Baum et al., 2008). During observation of these activities (i.e., making oatmeal, writing a check) initiation, execution (i.e., organization, sequencing, judgment and safety), and termination are scored. The administrator offers structured cues to facilitate task completion, which aids occupational therapists in determining the level of assistance that individuals will require to complete activities of daily living and instrumental activities of daily living in their natural environment. The Executive Function Performance Test was originally intended for use with stroke patients but has also been validated for use with substance-using homeless individuals with mental illness (Raphael-Greenfield, 2012).

Kettle Test

For patients who are likely to have experienced a head injury, the Kettle Test may be used to assess executive function (Hartman-Maeir et al., 2009). The Kettle Test is quick to perform and requires only a few inexpensive supplies. In this assessment, patients prepare a hot drink of their choice as well as a hot drink for the assessment administrator. Performance is scored for intact performance, slow performance, and type of cueing (e.g., general, specific, or physical assistance required). Although this assessment is not expressly intended for such, it also can give occupational therapists an opportunity to observe patients' safety awareness.

Interventions

In order to be supportive of community integration and the client being an agent of change in their own lives, it is absolutely essential that interventions are designed with the cooperation of the client and not prescribed to them. These interventions should always be created with discharge in mind for the same reasons. Allowing the client to self-determine can sometimes be the most difficult technique to master, however, but also one of the most essential. People who have lived highly structured lives in shelters or incarcerated, as well as for people who have lived in the moment-to-moment chaos of street homelessness, may not have had ample opportunity to practice independent, thoughtful decision making and problem solving. Our best learning, however, comes from making errors and then having to deal with the consequences. As practitioners, we often will feel the compulsion to protect our clients from negative outcomes of their choices. In this case, however, we must differentiate between a decision that truly endangers the client or others and behavior that we simply do not agree with or makes us worry. If we give in to that compulsion to rescue them, we are often denying them these essential opportunities for learning. That kind of "protection" can also be interpreted as judgment, which can harm the therapeutic relationship. For people in recovery from homelessness, trauma, and mental illness, it is key that they are able to develop resilience that lasts outside of the clinic and supports their eventual discharge. Therapeutic frameworks, such as Motivational Interviewing and the Transtheoretical Stages of Change, can be supportive of the therapist remaining in their role of the facilitator, and the client remaining in control of their own trajectory.

Discharge Planning

As individuals leave our care, it is important to think beyond cessation of services so that we are able to leave them with connections to further care, along with other varied tools they need to ensure a smooth transition into the next stage of their lives. Obtaining housing and/or employment may seem like an endpoint, but this is where the client's ability to maintain healthy routines and access services independently is really tested. If the occupational therapist has helped the client develop self-care and leisure routines to support wellness, social support networks, and a plan for accessing services as needed, the client is bound to succeed. Too often, however, these plans are not in place and a person may not be able to maintain their trajectory without structured support, which in turn leads to lost housing or employment. Income and subsidies are also essential to consider when thinking of discharge. If an individual receives Medicaid insurance, public assistance income, supplemental security income, and/or food stamps, occupational therapy can help the client to consider how housing or employment may change these benefits and what the implications may be. In a shelter, an individual receives a bed without paying rent and three meals a day free of charge. If 30% of their small income goes toward rent, there is very little money left to cover transportation and food, much less leisure or clothing. These are eventualities that can be overcome, but they do require careful planning in partnership with the client. Remember also that the recovery model is defined by stages of progression and regression. Helping a client remember this as they leave treatment can be facilitative of their returning to treatment as needed. A timely return to treatment can be the difference between lost housing, ruined relationships, and lost employment, and simply taking a break from the routine to process change, heal, and find support.

Tips and Advice From the Field

Finding Employment

Finding employment in emerging settings can be challenging. Seeking such a position is worth the effort, but it often requires creativity. In larger urban areas, occupational therapy in mental health is growing quickly. In others, therapists may be pioneers. The following are some tips for job searching:

- Participate in national and local occupational therapy association committees or groups that explore the community setting of choice (e.g., American Occupational Therapy Association Special Interest Sections, local mental health task force).
- Contact the university's fieldwork coordinator, previous clinical supervisors, and mental health professors. Having a recommendation or lead from an established professional in this area is valuable.
- Offer to supervise occupational therapy students from the local university in a site of interest. Setting up the placement requires much time and work, but occupational therapy is often the best advertisement for the profession. Many occupational therapists around the world have

been able to demonstrate the profession's unique value this way and then successfully advocate for permanent paid positions.

- When seeking positions, consider any role that an occupational therapist could fill and make a case. For instance, occupational therapy functions well in the vocational department of out-patient substance abuse treatment as many patients require training in foundational life skills before seeking employment and also ongoing support while being employed.

Continuing Education

Burgeoning mental health therapists can benefit from the recommendations given throughout Chapter 8 of this book and apply these to working in shelters, housing programs, substance use rehabilitation, prisons, and other emerging settings. Occupational therapists must maintain excellent professional boundaries, be flexible and adaptable, and study trauma-informed practice. These settings, however, may require some specialized knowledge.

- Occupational therapists in housing programs, shelters, and any other setting where patients are or have been homeless should familiarize themselves with local housing policies and the housing application process. Patients with cognitive impairment may require assistance from occupational therapy to complete the process, such as schedule or calendar creation and escorts to and from appointments. Interviewing and communication skills development may be required to prepare for housing interviews.
- Therapists in these settings should research consistent sources of free clothing, food, and hot meals as patients who cycle through institutional settings are often losing items or have them stolen. Patients either may not be aware that these services exist or do not know how to access them. Learning where local soup kitchens and clothing distribution points are is an efficient way of beginning the work of developing community integration.
- Therapists should understand the funding sources of the organization they work for and of similar organizations in the area. Funders can be federal, state, local, or private, with different program goals and requirements. As such, a developing occupational therapy practice may be shaped by these forces.

Understanding Personal Perspectives and Societal Forces

In addition to more formal study areas, occupational therapists working in this field should make an effort to understand the lived experiences and personal perspectives of their patients. There are numerous books and articles that chronicle the stories of those living in poverty, who are or have been homeless, who are or have been incarcerated, and who are struggling with substance use disorders. The following is a short reading list meant to inspire further research into specific practice areas and populations:

- *Grand Central Winter: Stories from the Street* by Lee Stringer (1998)
- *The Careless Society: Community and Its Counterfeits* by John McKnight (1995)
- *Nickel and Dimed: On (Not) Getting by in America* by Barbara Ehrenreich (2001)
- *The Body Keeps the Score: Brain, Mind, and Body in the Healing of Trauma* by Bessel van der Kolk (2014)
- *In the Realm of Hungry Ghosts: Close Encounters with Addiction* by Gabor Maté (2008)
- *Never Enough: The Neuroscience and Experience of Addiction* by Judith Grisel (2019)
- *Perspectives on Disability and Rehabilitation: Contesting Assumptions, Challenging Practice* by Karen Whalley Hammell (2006)

TABLE 13-4

Sample Goals and Interventions

SETTING	LONG-TERM GOAL EXAMPLES	SHORT-TERM GOAL EXAMPLES	OCCUPATIONS/ SKILLS TARGETED
Outpatient substance use treatment Length of participation ranges	"I want to have a healthy relationship with my daughter." Jim will stop using heroin daily.	Jim will attend and participate in the emotional regulation group to develop more coping skills. Jim will explore several new activities with occupational therapy to begin building a healthy leisure routine as boredom can contribute to substance use. Jim will participate in a journaling club to develop self-awareness, specifically of triggers and responses. Jim will research and begin attending a range of local support group meetings to begin building social support outside the treatment facility.	Emotional regulation skills Leisure participation Self-awareness skills Social skills Social support building
Homeless shelter Length of participation ranges	"I want to move out of the shelter into an apartment." Samantha will successfully secure subsidized tenancy with assistance from occupational therapist and case manager.	Samantha will retrieve copies of her Social Security card, birth certificate, and driver's license. Samantha will attend her weekly housing meeting and will arrive on time. Samantha will practice interview skills (verbal and nonverbal presentation) to prepare for housing interviews. Samantha will apply for membership in a local mental health clubhouse to build social support, which will mediate loneliness after moving.	Community integration Organization Time management Consequential thinking Communication skills Social skills Leisure participation Health management

(continued)

TABLE 13-4 (CONTINUED)

Sample Goals and Interventions

SETTING	LONG-TERM GOAL EXAMPLES	SHORT-TERM GOAL EXAMPLES	OCCUPATIONS/ SKILLS TARGETED
Housing First program Permanent housing	"I want to stay here and just live a normal life: go to the store, have a girlfriend, and invite my family over for dinner." Monroe will maintain a healthy daily routine that supports maintenance of health, home, relationships, and employment.	Monroe will participate in weekly cooking groups to learn healthy recipes that can be prepared using inexpensive ingredients. Monroe will explore resources at his local library (e.g., computers, books, DVDs, classes, clubs) to develop a leisure routine, as well as a natural social support network. Monroe will research local mental and physical health care providers (with assistance) to maintain his well-being. Monroe will create and follow a budget that includes leisure activities as well as necessities.	Food preparation Food safety Organization Consequential thinking Planning Community integration Leisure participation Social support building Health management Coping skills Money management

- *Occupational Experiences of Homelessness: A Systematic Review and Meta-Aggregation* by Carrie Anne Marshall et al. (2019)
- *Bridging the Transition From Homeless to Housed: A Social Justice Framework to Guide the Practice of Occupational Therapists* by Carrie Anne Marshall et al. (2020)

Sample goals and interventions are presented in Table 13-4.

Suitability for Practice

The lives of people experiencing a mélange of discrimination, homelessness, health and social disparities, mental illness, and physical disability take many forms with many stops and starts along the way. How histories, barriers, and strengths fit together and contribute to the recovery of each individual is unique. As such, a flexible occupational therapy practice that is patient driven and focused on meeting the person "where they are" to work toward personally relevant goals will likely be most effective. Whereas certain curricula and protocols can be helpful in these settings, they are not inclusive. The recommendations in this chapter are intended to be a starting point, not a prescription.

References

Aurand, A., Emmanuel, D., Threet, D., Rafi, I., & Yentel, D. (2020). *The gap: A shortage of affordable homes.* National Low Income Housing Coalition. https://reports.nlihc.org/sites/default/files/gap/Gap-Report_2020.pdf

Barnes, S. M., Russell, L. M., Hostetter, T. A., Forster, J. E., Devore, M. D., & Brenner, L. A. (2015). Characteristics of traumatic brain injuries sustained among veterans seeking homeless services. *Journal of Health Care for the Poor and Underserved, 26,* 92–105. https://doi.org/10.1353/hpu.2015.0010

Baum, C. M., Connor, L. T., Morrison, T., Hahn, M., Dromerick, A. W., & Edwards, D. F. (2008). Reliability, validity, and clinical utility of the Executive Function Performance Test: A measure of executive function in a sample of people with stroke. *American Journal of Occupational Therapy, 62*(4), 446–455. https://doi.org/10.5014/ajot.62.4.446

Centers for Disease Control and Prevention. (2019). Symptoms of traumatic brain injury (TBI). https://www.cdc.gov/traumaticbraininjury/symptoms.html

Dams-O'Connor, K., Cantor, J. B., Brown, M., Dijkers, M. P., Spielman, L. A., & Gordon, W. A. (2014). Screening for traumatic brain injury: Findings and public health implications. *Journal of Head Trauma Rehabilitation, 29,* 479–489. https://doi.org/10.1097/HTR.0000000000000099

Doig, E., Fleming, J., Kuipers, P., & Cornwell, P. L. (2010). Clinical utility of the combined use of the Canadian Occupational Performance Measure and Goal Attainment Scaling. *American Journal of Occupational Therapy, 64,* 904–914. https://doi.org/10.5014/ajot.2010.08156

Ehrenreich, B. (2001). *Nickel and dimed: On (not) getting by in America.* Metropolitan Books.

Goering, P., Veldhuizen, S., Watson, A., Adair, C., Kopp, B., Latimer, E., Nelson, G., MacNaughton, E., Streiner, D., & Aubry, T. (2014). National At Home/Chez Soi final report. *Mental Health Commission of Canada.* http://www.mentalhealthcommission.ca

Grisel, J. (2019). *Never enough: The neuroscience and experience of addiction.* Anchor Books.

Hammell, K. W. (2006). *Perspectives on disability and rehabilitation: Contesting assumptions, challenging practice.* Elsevier Health Sciences.

Hartman-Maeir, A., Harel, H., & Katz, N. (2009). Kettle Test—A brief measure of cognitive functional performance: Reliability and validity in stroke rehabilitation. *American Journal of Occupational Therapy, 63*(5), 592–599. https://doi.org/10.5014/ajot.63.5.592

Hawk, M., Coulter, R. W., Egan, J. E., Fisk, S., Friedman, M. R., Tula, M., & Kinsky, S. (2017). Harm reduction principles for healthcare settings. *Harm Reduction Journal, 14*(1), 70. https://doi.org/10.1186/s12954-017-0196-4

Law, M. C., Baptiste, S., Carswell, A., McColl, M. A., Polatajko, H. J., & Pollock, N. (2014). *Canadian Occupational Performance Measure (COPM)* (4th ed.). CAOT Publications ACE.

Marshall, C. A., Boland, L., Westover, L. A., Wickett, S., Roy, L., Mace, J., Gequrtz, R., & Kirsh, B. (2019). Occupational experiences of homelessness: A systematic review and meta-aggregation. *Scandinavian Journal of Occupational Therapy, 27*(6), 1–14. https://doi.org/10.1080/11038128.2019.1689292

Marshall, C. A., Gewurtz, R., Barbic, S., Roy, L., Lysaght, R., Ross, C., Becker, A., Cooke, A., & Kirsh, B. (2020). *Bridging the transition from homeless to housed: A social justice framework to guide the practice of occupational therapists.* https://www.sjmhlab.com/publications

Maté, G. (2008). *In the realm of hungry ghosts: Close encounters with addiction.* North Atlantic Books.

McKnight, J. (1995). *The careless society: Community and its counterfeits.* Basic Books.

Raphael-Greenfield, E. (2012). Assessing executive and community functioning among homeless persons with substance use disorders using the Executive Function Performance Test. *Occupational Therapy International, 19*(3), 135–143. https://doi.org/10.1002/oti.1328

Stringer, L. (1998). *Grand central winter.* Simon and Schuster.

Stubbs, J. L., Thornton, A. E., Sevick, J. M., Silverberg, N. D., Barr, A. M., Honer, W. G., & Panenka, W. J. (2020). Traumatic brain injury in homeless and marginally housed individuals: A systematic review and meta-analysis. *Lancet Public Health, 5*(1), E19–E32. https://doi.org/10.1016/S2468-2667(19)30188-4

Substance Abuse and Mental Health Services Administration. (2012). *SAMHSA's working definition of recovery.* https://store.samhsa.gov/system/files/pep12-recdef.pdf

U.S. Department of Health and Human Services Centers for Disease Control and Prevention. (2007). *Traumatic brain injury in prisons and jails: An unrecognized problem.* https://stacks.cdc.gov/view/cdc/11668

U.S. Department of Housing and Urban Development. (2020). *The 2019 Annual Homeless Assessment Report (AHAR) to Congress.* https://files.hudexchange.info/resources/documents/2019-AHAR-Part-1.pdf

U.S. Department of Housing and Urban Development. (n.d.). *Housing First in permanent supportive housing.* https://files.hudexchange.info/resources/documents/Housing-First-Permanent-Supportive-Housing-Brief.pdf

U.S. Interagency Council on Homelessness. (2018). *Homelessness in America: Focus on veterans.* https://www.usich.gov/resources/uploads/asset_library/Homelessness_in_America._Focus_on_Veterans.pdf

Van der Kolk, B. A. (2014). *The body keeps the score: Brain, mind, and body in the healing of trauma.* Penguin Books.

Wong, Y. L. I., & Solomon, P. L. (2002). Community integration of persons with psychiatric disabilities in supportive independent housing: A conceptual model and methodological considerations. *Mental Health Services Research, 4*(1), 13–28. https://doi.org/10.1023/a:1014093008857

Yohanna, D. (2013). Deinstitutionalization of people with mental illness: Causes and consequences. *AMA Journal of Ethics, 15*(10), 886–891. https://doi.org/10.1001/virtualmentor.2013.15.10.mhst1-1310

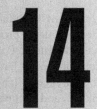

14

Literacy Across the Lifespan

Mindy Garfinkel, OTD, OTR/L, ATP

Literacy in a Nutshell

Occupational therapy practice has evolved over time to meet the ever-changing needs of individuals, groups, and society. Whereas the *Occupational Therapy Practice Framework, Fourth Edition* (American Occupational Therapy Association [AOTA], 2020) guides practice, the scope of practice within the *Occupational Therapy Practice Framework, Fourth Edition* has expanded to include new and innovative practice areas to meet societal needs and remain relevant in today's world.

Literacy is embedded in culture and daily lives. Consider the consequences of being a non-reader in a public school setting. What would happen to a rider on public transportation unable to read the subway map? How would a patient self-administer medication appropriately if they could not read the medicine bottle? How would an individual apply for food stamps if unable to complete the language-rich application?

Traditionally, *literacy* has been defined as the ability to read and write (Cambridge University Press, n.d.; Merriam-Webster, n.d.). However, contemporary theorists have broadened this definition, noting that perceptions of what literacy entails are complex and varied, as people create meaning not only from written words but also from spoken language, culture, and life experiences. Literacy helps individuals derive meaning from experiences and environment, facilitating the ability to engage in meaningful daily occupations and interactions with others (Alberta Government, n.d.; Grajo & Gutman, 2019b).

Akselrud, R. (Ed.). *Quintessential Occupational Therapy:*
A Guide to Areas of Practice (pp 157-165).
© 2023 Taylor & Francis Group.

The concept of *functional literacy* has been introduced to identify literacy as the process through which individuals decode written language, process it, and use it to perform various occupations, such as self-care, to support independence within communities and society (Grajo & Gutman, 2019b). These expanded visions of literacy have created opportunities for a variety of professionals, such as educators, psychologists, speech–language pathologists, assistive technology specialists, vocational rehabilitation specialists, and occupational therapy practitioners, to become integral members of the literacy team.

Occupational Therapy's Role

When viewed through the lens of function and occupational performance, the distinct value of occupational therapy in support of individuals with literacy challenges can be seen with greater clarity. For example, occupational therapists have been trained to address early literacy skills and other critical skill components that may act as barriers to engagement using play (AOTA, n.d.a). Furthermore, therapists have been trained to analyze activities within the context of the environment, distinctly preparing them to adapt and modify activities and environments as needed to make literacy-rich experiences more accessible and engaging for individuals, groups, and populations.

Individuals who have difficulty decoding and processing written language typically have been diagnosed with a medical or skill impairment or may have been deprived of opportunities to engage in literacy-rich experiences (Table 14-1).

Evaluation and Assessments

Occupational therapists perform a comprehensive evaluation to determine the need for and intensity of services. Literacy assessments typically begin with observations in the natural environments where literacy-related occupations are performed (e.g., in a restaurant when reading a menu, in class during a math lesson). Knowledge of performance skills in areas required for literacy-based occupations is needed to identify barriers and facilitators to participation and engagement.

For literacy, standardized evaluations are administered for vision, motor performance, cognition, behavior, and sensory integration skills. In addition, literacy-specific assessments include the Inventory of Reading Occupations–Pediatric Version (Grajo et al., 2019) and the Inventory of Reading Occupations–Adult Version (Grajo & Gutman, 2019a). Several handwriting evaluations target written output, such as the Evaluation Tool of Children's Handwriting (Amundson, 1995) and the Detailed Assessment of Speed of Handwriting (Barnett et al., 2007). Age-appropriate and context-specific occupation-based assessments can be completed to create a more comprehensive occupational profile from which practitioners can develop goals and intervention plans.

Interventions

Service Delivery Models

Literacy-based interventions use a variety of service delivery models on the basis of the needs identified through the evaluation, a comprehensive environmental analysis, and an activity analysis. For example, a college student introduced to "talking" software for the first time might initially receive their direct intervention in a private conference room rather than in their classroom where the instruction might disturb others. However, once the student has mastered the program outside of the classroom, it is appropriate for them to receive their intervention in the classroom to facilitate generalization to the natural environment.

Literacy-based interventions can be one-on-one or provided in small group settings (e.g., reading groups). Whereas direct interventions can take place in a variety of contexts, research has shown that the most effective service delivery models are contextually based (Bazyk & Cahill, 2014; Garfinkel & Seruya, 2018; Handley-More et al., 2013; Polichino & Jackson, 2014; Silverman, 2011; Watt & Richards, 2016).

TABLE 14-1

Variables Creating a Risk for Literacy-Related Challenges

DIAGNOSIS	SKILLS DEFICIT AREA	LIMITED ACCESS TO RESOURCES
Vision impairment	Visual perception	Children of parents who are illiterate
Hearing impairment	Executive functioning	Individuals who are homeless
Cognitive impairment or brain injury	Motor performance and coordination	Individuals who are incarcerated
Developmental disability	Praxis or motor planning	Individuals living in poverty
Learning disability	Behavioral regulation	Victims of neglect
Attention-deficit/ hyperactivity disorder	Sensory integration	Individuals for whom English is not their primary language
Autism spectrum disorder	Emotional regulation	Nursing home residents
Speech and language impairment	Communication	Immigrants without permanent residency status

Interventions also can occur indirectly, wherein occupational therapists provide services on behalf of patients or students. For example, therapists might intervene with a single patient by collaborating with their daughter to discuss medication management or might work on behalf of groups or populations by providing training on the use of sensory-based strategies in the classroom to improve students' attention before writing activities.

In response to societal needs, occupational therapy intervention sometimes occurs virtually via a telehealth model (see Chapter 16 in this book). Using this model is helpful for individuals who reside in remote areas where they do not have access to therapists and also allows practitioners to see individuals in their natural environments (AOTA, 2018b).

The frequency and duration of occupational therapy interventions are varied on the basis of the needs within the context of the environment. For example, a nursing home resident who is nonverbal due to a recent traumatic brain injury may be seen daily for 15 minutes in the morning to help them fill out their daily menu. A teenager learning to use assistive technology may require frequent direct intervention for a month, followed by indirect intervention in which the therapist collaborates monthly with the team to support them in a variety of settings.

Public Health Approaches

Many occupational therapists use a public health approach in their practice, focusing on health promotion for groups or populations to prevent the need for more intensive services later and to support independence in daily life. A variety of applications are available that use picture schedules, eliminating the need to rely on written language, thus helping individuals be more independent in their daily occupations. For example, using a public health approach, practitioners can educate family members and caregivers of individuals living with developmental disabilities about the use of everyday technology and applications to support independence (Garfinkel, 2019; Golisz et al., 2018).

Universal Design for Learning

Universal Design for Learning (UDL) is a "framework to improve and optimize teaching and learning for all people based on scientific insights into how humans learn" (CAST, 2020, p. 1). UDL applies the principles of equal access, flexibility, simplicity, and efficiency to both the environment and the process of teaching and learning, frequently through the use of mainstream and specialized technology (Post, 2015). For example, using a UDL model, individuals with visual deficits may be offered books on tape to access the curricular materials through auditory rather than visual means.

Multi-Tiered Systems of Support

The Multi-Tiered Systems of Support education framework identifies students at risk in academic or behavioral areas and provides them with team-based tiered interventions on the basis of the intensity of their needs (Cahill, 2019). Using this evidence-based model, practitioners collaborate with stakeholders to develop whole school programming that benefits students with varying educational needs. For example, interventions can include offering a "mindful moment" after the morning pledge, in which the entire school is led in a 5-minute meditation before the school day commences, or movement breaks, which are strategically implemented throughout the school day to foster appropriate alertness levels in all students.

Intervention Categories

Interventions in literacy fall under three broad categories: habilitation and rehabilitation, adaptation and modification, and advocacy.

Habilitation and Rehabilitation

Habilitation and rehabilitation interventions help individuals learn new or relearn skills that may have been lost or impaired (AOTA, 2018a). Examples include the following:

- Using multisensory materials (e.g., PlayDoh [Hasbro], shaving cream, stencils) to teach correct letter formation.
- Singing alphabet songs while playing on the playground.
- Cutting out letters from a magazine to create words.
- Highlighting targeted letters, words, or numbers on a menu.
- Completing a word search puzzle.

Adaptation and Modification

Adaptation and modification interventions target revision of the activity or environment to increase level of independence (AOTA, 2020). Examples include the following:

- Helping patients learn how to write emails using speech-to-text software.
- Teaching students to use a blank piece of paper to cover part of a page so that they can visually focus on the exposed portion of the page.
- Teaching individuals to increase the font size on their iPad (Apple).
- Helping workers construct an ergonomically correct workspace with supportive seating and a computer screen that aligns with their line of vision.
- Teaching students to use graph paper when completing math problems to help them maintain number columns.

Advocacy

Advocacy interventions promote occupational justice and individuals' empowerment to find resources to support full participation in daily life occupations (AOTA, 2020). Examples include the following:

- Collaborating with a patient's physician to write a letter to their insurance provider justifying the need for a switch that will allow them to use an augmentative communication device independently.
- Asking a teacher to print the homework assignments on the board rather than writing them in cursive so that the entire class will have an easier time reading them.
- Giving a Spanish-speaking patient an index card that says "I need an interpreter" so that they may present it when needed at pharmacies and physician offices.
- Coaching a college student through the process of visiting the Office of Accessibility to inquire about any accommodations they might be eligible to receive.
- Contacting elected representatives or starting a petition to make a neighborhood park more inclusive by installing Braille signage.

Role of Assistive Technology

Assistive technology can be used to help students and patients gain access to and increase their engagement in a variety of literacy-rich occupations. Examples include software that converts text to speech and speech to text, tape recorders, and positioning devices. Assistive technology can provide a method through which individuals can make social connections (e.g., social media platforms, email, texting, gaming). Augmentative communication devices and specialized applications can provide some nonverbal individuals with a "voice."

Furthermore, assistive technology aligns with the public health approach. Assistive technology can support *all* individuals through common accessibility features on most mobile and laptop devices and frequently uses a multimodal method of presenting information.

Matching the appropriate assistive technology to individuals involves careful consideration of their factors, the environments within which they will be using the device, the occupations that the device will be supporting, and the characteristics of the technology itself (Cook et al., 2020; Zabala, 2005). Collaborating with users and other stakeholders when deciding on appropriate assistive technology recommendations is the preferred method of gaining a more holistic perspective of the user and preventing the device's abandonment of use.

As technology evolves and user needs change, the evaluation and reevaluation process is ongoing. Whenever possible, the expertise of a professional certified in assistive technology (ATP) should be sought. Many ATPs are occupational therapy practitioners who have received their certification through the Rehabilitation Engineering and Assistive Technology Society of North America (RESNA); however, other health care professionals also may have RESNA certification and expertise in this area (RESNA, 2022).

Intervention Settings

Literacy-based intervention is viewed most often as occurring in school settings because a main student occupation is to learn reading and writing skills. However, as occupational therapy intervention in support of literacy occurs across the lifespan, therapists can infuse literacy-based interventions into most settings.

Discharge Planning and Transitioning

The discharge planning objective is to determine the appropriate setting for the client to transition to when goals are met. It can also include client and caregiver education regarding adaptation techniques, utilization of equipment, and environmental modifications. The overarching goal of discharge planning is maintenance, restoration, and promoting wellness. Transition planning involves a referral to an occupational therapist or provider from another profession. Transition planning can be for transitioning from one stage to another, like a student transitioning from junior high to high school. Transition planning also includes transitioning from a set of needs to an alternative set of needs, like an older adult in a falls prevention program transitioning to a community exercise program (AOTA, 2020).

Tips and Advice From the Field

Caseload and Schedule

Occupational therapy practitioners are hired directly by a school or facility or through a contract agency. Hours and caseload sizes typically depend on student and patient needs and those of the facility. However, employment, hours, and caseload size may affect the availability to engage in a public health approach, which often is not reimbursed by third-party payers (Table 14-2).

A Successful Case

For several years, while working in a public elementary school, I (M.G.) collaborated with the team members supporting one self-contained classroom of kindergarten and first grade students to provide weekly cooking classes. In addition to myself, the team included the classroom teacher, who was certified in special education, a speech–language pathologist, and classroom assistants. A maximum of 12 students were in each class. All students had educational disabilities, and most received either direct or indirect occupational therapy services.

As part of the program, the team members met weekly to plan food-based activities that aligned with the classroom's literacy-based themes. For example, when the class was reading *Brown Bear, Brown Bear* (Martin & Carle, 1987), we made "Teddy Bear Toast" using whole-wheat toast, cream cheese, bananas, and blueberries. Recipes were continually revised considering students' food allergies, sensory needs, strengths, and challenges. Each group followed a protocol that we developed jointly:

- We read the book together.
- We reviewed the recipe, which was written on a large easel, using as few words as possible and supplementing the recipe with pictures.
- We placed all food items and cooking utensils on a separate table, and because the recipe was being read as a group, we assigned students to locate the items on that table and bring them to the "cooking table."
- Each team member used their expertise to support the students, addressing individualized education plan goals while preparing the food.
- The class ate the finished product together while discussing what the students liked or did not like about the activity.

From this highly successful literacy-based group that was interdisciplinary and collaborative, I took away the importance of listening and learning from other team members, who each have a distinct voice. Over the 10 years that I have been involved with the group, the vast majority of students were highly engaged in all aspects of the activities, and the therapeutic interventions occurred within the context of their natural environment, the classroom, during snack time.

Suitability for Practice

Experienced occupational therapists likely have been incorporating literacy-based intervention into practice without putting a name to it. However, therapists are encouraged to be more mindful of ways in which to enrich practice by providing access for patients and students to occupations that

TABLE 14-2

Literacy-Based Intervention Settings and Goals

SETTING	SAMPLE INTERVENTION	GOAL
Early intervention in the home	Coaching parents on how to read to their child	Within 1 month, J.P.'s parents will read picture books to him before bed, following the suggested guidelines by the occupational therapist, on five of seven occasions.
Private practice	Using sensory-based strategies to change alertness levels to facilitate availability for literacy-based activities	Within 6 months, J.P. will use sensory-based strategies before engaging in writing tasks in the classroom, on four of five occasions, with minimal visual cueing.
Public or private school	Educating students and staff about accessibility features on tablets, laptop computers, and desktop computers	Within 1 month, all staff members in the self-contained classroom will use Google accessibility features on their Chromebooks to change font sizes for students with visual impairments, 80% of the time.
Hospital	Advocating for an interpreter and written materials in patient's primary language	Within 2 months, home programs written in Spanish will be made available and distributed to Spanish-speaking patients at discharge, 100% of the time.
Inpatient rehabilitation	Collaborating with the patient's speech-language pathologist to obtain and train them to use an augmentative communication device	Within 1 month, the patient will use their augmentative communication device to order two of their three daily meals, with 80% accuracy, each day.
Skilled-nursing facility	Collaborating with the team members to obtain a wheelchair seating system for a resident with poor postural control, so that they may explore their literacy-rich environment and be appropriately positioned to engage in literacy-based activities	Within 6 months, the resident will sit supported in their wheelchair for 30 minutes while playing Bingo, once per week, with the other residents on their floor, without complaint of discomfort or evidence of skin breakdown, 100% of the time.
Prison system	Advocating for reading materials in the primary language of incarcerated individuals and for materials that span a variety of literacy levels	Within 9 months, individuals will be able to access materials at their reading level from the prison library on three of five occasions.

Table 14-3

Areas to Review to Prepare for Engagement in Literacy-Related Interventions

PRACTICE AREA	AREA TO REVIEW	RATIONALE
Schools	Common Core state standards	To learn what is expected of students in the curriculum
Schools	Multi-tiered system of supports UDL	To learn about public health models used in school-based practice
Schools	Developmental milestones	To help recognize typical from atypical development
All practice areas	Evidence-based articles and literacy resources	To support the use of evidence-based practice
All practice areas	Sensory-based strategies to optimize alertness levels	To increase student availability for instruction and intervention
All practice areas	State and federal legislation	To learn about the laws governing this practice area
All practice areas	Assistive technology to support literacy	To keep current with technological advances in this area

may be inherently literacy rich. New graduates and clinicians who are changing practice areas are strongly encouraged to adopt this emerging niche in all practice areas.

Occupational therapists working in this niche must be able to collaborate with a variety of stakeholders across settings. Therefore, therapists should be effective spoken and written communicators. Therapists should be creative and able to understand and support others' perspectives when problem solving. Therapists should have a strong sense of what occupational therapy is and how literacy fits into the scope of practice because they will need this knowledge when advocating for the profession's distinct role in support of literacy.

Supports to the Adoption of This Practice Area

Occupational therapists interested in incorporating literacy into their practice should seek resources and mentorship opportunities within or outside their schools or facilities. It may be efficacious to partner with an ATP if considering using assistive technology as part of the intervention. A powerful resource for obtaining resources and locating mentors is AOTA's (2019) Literacy Community of Practice. AOTA members can join this group of like-minded individuals who meet virtually once per month to learn more about the distinct role of occupational therapy in support of literacy and to disseminate resources. Because occupational therapists address literacy across the lifespan, it is important to review several areas in preparation for providing literacy-based interventions (Table 14-3).

References

Alberta Government. (n.d.). *Literacy* [Fact Sheet]. https://education.alberta.ca/media/3402193/lit-fact-sheet.pdf

American Occupational Therapy Association. (n.d.). *Literacy.* https://www.aota.org/Practice/Children-Youth/literacy.aspx

American Occupational Therapy Association. (2018a). *New coding requirement for billing habilitative and re-habilitative services in some private insurance plans.* https://www.aota.org/advocacy/advocacy-news/2018/new-coding-requirement-for-billing-habilitative-rehabilitative-services

American Occupational Therapy Association. (2018b). Telehealth in occupational therapy. *American Journal of Occupational Therapy, 72*(Suppl. 2), 7212410059p1-7212410059p18. https://doi.org/10.5014/ajot.2018.72S219

American Occupational Therapy Association. (2019). *Literacy community of practice (CoP).* https://www.aota.org/~/media/Corporate/Files/Practice/Manage/SIS/cop/Literacy-Infographic-communities-of-practice-2019.pdf

American Occupational Therapy Association. (2020). Occupational therapy practice framework: Domain and process (4th ed.). *American Journal of Occupational Therapy, 74*(Suppl. 2), 7412410010p1-7412410010p87. https://doi.org/10.5014/ajot.2020.74S2001

Amundson, S. J. (1995). *Evaluation tool of children's handwriting.* https://www.therapro.com/Browse-Category/Handwriting-Evaluations/Evaluation-Tool-of-Childrens-Handwriting-ETCH.html

Barnett, A., Henderson, S. E., Scheib, B., & Schulz, J. (2007). *Detailed assessment of speed of handwriting (DASH).* Pearson.

Bazyk, S., & Cahill, S. (2014). School-based occupational therapy. In J. Case-Smith & J. C. O'Brien (Eds.), *Occupational therapy for children and adolescents* (7th ed., pp. 664–703). Mosby.

Cahill, S. M. (2019). Best practices in multi-tiered systems of support. In G. F. Clark, J. E. Rioux, & B. E. Chandler (Eds.), *Best practices for occupational therapy in schools* (2nd ed., pp. 211-217). AOTA Press.

Cambridge University Press. (n.d.). *Definition of literacy.* https://dictionary.cambridge.org/dictionary/english/literacy

CAST. (2020). Universal design for learning. http://www.cast.org/our-work/about-udl.html#.Xh8g4chKg2w

Cook, A. M., Polgar, J. M., & Encarnação, P. (2020). *Assistive technologies: Principles & practice* (5th ed., pp.1-14). Elsevier.

Garfinkel, M. (2019). *Everyday technologies to support independence in instrumental activities of daily living.* Westchester ARC Technology Conference, Dobbs Ferry, NY, United States.

Garfinkel, M., & Seruya, F. M. (2018). Therapists' perceptions of the 3:1 Service Delivery Model: A workload approach to school-based practice. *Journal of Occupational Therapy, Schools, & Early Intervention, 11*(3), 273–290. https://doi.org/10.1080/19411243.2018.1455551

Golisz, K., Waldman-Levi, A., Swierat, R. P., & Toglia, J. (2018). Adults with intellectual disabilities: Case studies using everyday technology to support daily living skills. *British Journal of Occupational Therapy, 81*(9), 514–524. https://doi.org/10.1177/0308022618764781

Grajo, L., Candler, C., Bowyer, P., Schultz, S., & Thomson, J. (2019). The inventory of reading occupations—Pediatric version. https://www.ps.columbia.edu/education/academic-programs/programs-occupational-therapy/faculty-innovations/ot-literacy

Grajo, L., & Gutman, S. (2019a). The inventory of reading occupations—Adult version. https://www.ps.columbia.edu/education/academic-programs/programs-occupational-therapy/faculty-innovations/ot-literacy

Grajo, L. C., & Gutman, S. A. (2019b). The role of occupational therapy in functional literacy. *Open Journal of Occupational Therapy, 7*(1), 1–9. https://doi.org/10.15453/2168-6408.1511

Handley-More, D., Wall, E., Orentlicher, M. L., & Hollenbeck, J. (2013). Working in early intervention and school settings: Current views of best practice. *Early Intervention & School Special Interest Section Quarterly, 20*(2), 1–4.

Martin, B., & Carle, E. (1987). *Brown Bear, Brown Bear.* Penguin.

Merriam-Webster (n.d.). *Definition of literacy.* https://www.merriam-webster.com/dictionary/literacy

Polichino, J. E., & Jackson, L. (2014). *Frequently asked questions: Transforming caseload to workload in school-based occupational therapy services.* http://www.aota.org/-/media/Corporate/Files/Secure/Practice/Children/Workload-fact.pdf

Post, K. M. (2015). *Occupational therapy and universal design for learning* [Fact sheet]. https://www.aota.org/~/media/Corporate/Files/AboutOT/Professionals/WhatIsOT/CY/Fact-Sheets/UDL%20fact%20sheet.pdf

Rehabilitation Engineering and Assistive Technology Society of North America. (2022). *About.* https://www.resna.org

Silverman, F. (2011). Promoting inclusion with occupational therapy: A coteaching model. *Journal of Occupational Therapy, Schools, & Early Intervention, 4*(2), 100–107. https://doi.org/10.1080/19411243.2011.595308

Watt, H., & Richards, L. G. (2016). Factors influencing occupational therapy practitioners' use of push-in and pull-out service delivery models in the school system [Poster presentation]. *American Journal of Occupational Therapy, 70*(Suppl. 1), 7011510205p1. https://doi.org/10.5014/ajot.2016.70S1-PO3068

Zabala, J. S. (2005). *Using the SETT Framework to level the learning field for students with disabilities.* Academia. http://www.joyzabala.com/uploads/Zabala_SETT_Leveling_the_Learning_Field.pdf

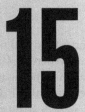

Holistic
Occupational Therapy

Anna Wold, OTR/L
and Miriam Wachspress, MS, OTR/L

Holistic Occupational Therapy in a Nutshell

Holistic occupational therapy is an emerging field that incorporates alternative therapies into professional practice. Holistic occupational therapists use mind–body–spirit modalities to treat the whole person, not just the presenting symptoms (Lubas & Vadnais, 2014).

Occupational Therapy's Role

Holistic occupational therapists can work in any setting—mental health, geriatric, outpatient, and pediatric. Their primary role is to work in a traditional therapy environment offering creative holistic solutions and techniques to help patients reach their goals. Because general Western culture has become more holistic focused, most "traditional" occupational therapists already may be incorporating holistic skills into their interventions without labeling themselves as "holistic."

The *Occupational Therapy Practice Framework, Fourth Edition* (American Occupational Therapy Association, 2020) encourages clinicians to look for holistic means of intervention, that is, to not only see the main diagnoses but also to examine other factors (e.g., social, environmental) that may be impeding progress. Occupational therapy is a holistic profession as it can assist a person with all aspects of their life.

Akselrud, R. (Ed.). *Quintessential Occupational Therapy:*
A Guide to Areas of Practice (pp 167-170).
© 2023 Taylor & Francis Group.

Evaluation and Assessments

Occupational therapists use both standardized and nonstandardized assessments, and holistic therapists more often use nonstandardized. Whereas standardized assessments examine patients' simple limiting factors to their functional abilities, nonstandardized assessments often provide more global or holistic information about subtle factors that may be impeding progress.

For example, for a patient with neck pain, a standardized assessment will show the limiting active range of motion and any functional difficulties. A nonstandardized assessment may focus on a patient's overall quality of life and thus indicate that bad work habits are causing them to overly flex their neck. A holistic therapist can recommend and educate a patient about better work habits and posture to help resolve any neck limitations.

Sample Interview

An occupational therapy patient interview might begin with the main complaints; however, the interview also can include questions that are seemingly unrelated to a patient's main concerns. For example, a holistic therapist working in orthopedics will ask if a patient with back pain also has pain in other areas of the body because often pain in one part of the body directly affects another. The therapist can use craniosacral therapy to treat the back pain, which also may relieve the neck pain.

Another component to explore in the interview is the patient's life, including eating, exercising, and sleeping. Often helping patients manage their stress can greatly improve their main complaints. For example, for a patient with back pain, the holistic therapist might ask about the sleep quality to see if they are sleeping enough and in a supportive posture.

Typical Interventions

The term *holistic* is general. It is hard to pinpoint typical diagnoses seen or skills addressed by holistic therapists because they offer a range of knowledge and techniques that can help most patients. For example, holistic therapists with training in craniosacral therapy can work in an outpatient facility with patients with limited active range of motion and pain in their back, neck, or upper extremities. Therapists with training in holistic stress management techniques (e.g., deep breathing, essential oils) can work in a mental health unit. Using their holistic knowledge with diagnoses, such as depression, bipolar disorder, and schizophrenia, they can teach patients how to utilize different breathing techniques to help manage stress during instrumental activities of daily living, such as maintaining a job. Therapists with yoga training can work in a pediatric setting, offering poses to children with low tone or poor sequencing or motor-planning skills. Using a client-centered measurement model instead of traditional methods can help in identifying the just-right challenge for the client. It can provide a basis for developing interventions that are specific to the client (Velozo, 2021).

Occupational therapy is uniquely positioned to address self-management from a holistic perspective, taking into account a client's intrinsic factors (cognitive, psychological, physical, sensory, emotional, and spiritual) and extrinsic influences (culture, social determinants of health, social support and capital, the built and natural environment, and policy) while considering the roles and activities in which the client participates (Fields & Smallfield, 2022).

Yoga

Yoga is a common form of exercise and relaxation across all ages and cultures. Through poses, breathing techniques, and postures, one can relax and strengthen various parts of the body. Yoga poses can be used with children with low tone, attention-deficit/hyperactivity disorder, and sensory-processing disorder. A modified yoga program using a chair can be used with older adults who have generalized weakness, gait instability, and neck or back pain. Other modifications and mobility devices can lead to improved confidence and decreased possibility of falling. Yoga is great for home exercise programs as well because it can be modified for body type and age to present the just-right challenge and be effective in improving strength and coordination (Velozo, 2021).

Breathing Techniques

Occupational therapists incorporate breathing techniques for before, during, and after activities. Breathing properly and easily can reduce heart rate, increase oxygen to the organs, and aid in relaxation. Education in breathing can come from yoga, meditation, and respiratory therapy. Because occupational therapists treat patients after having COVID-19, the importance of education about respiration and breathing is crucial to this new practice area.

Mothers and Infants

Occupational therapists can receive additional training for childbirth education, doula, lactation, and craniosacral therapy to aid women and infants before and after birth. Therapists can evaluate the functioning of mothers and their children in their activities of daily living and respective roles. Many therapists treat infants who have limitations in their oral musculature, offering various exercises and craniosacral therapy to aid in healing before and after surgery.

Craniosacral Therapy

Craniosacral therapy is a gentle touch that balances out the cerebrospinal fluid from the cranium (skull) to the sacrum (pelvis). Studies of the Upledger Institute International (2022) have suggested this therapy for almost any diagnosis, including autism spectrum disorder, attention-deficit/hyperactivity disorder, back pain, headaches, torticollis, and oral musculature limitations. Holistic occupational therapists can use craniosacral therapy to decrease muscle tension and pain.

Discharge Planning

Deeming the most suitable setting for a client for transition to maintain wellness is the main goal of discharge planning. The discharge planning process also includes client and caregiver education and referrals for continuing services. In addition, transition planning consists of transitioning from a set of needs to another set of needs. An example would be an older adult in a falls prevention program who is in the process of transitioning to a community exercise program (American Occupational Therapy Association, 2020).

Tips and Advice From the Field

Practitioners should consider which holistic approaches align with their current client base. Deep breathing and yoga, for example, may be helpful with most populations. It is critical for practitioners to lead by example, which involves understanding their own passions and motivations and using them in ways that can benefit the clients with whom they work. Practitioners interested should find their passion, take continuing education courses, and seek advice from others already in the field.

Typical Caseload and Workload

The workload is the same for more traditional and holistic therapists, only the lens that each type uses is different. For example, in rehabilitation, holistic therapists use traditional orthopedic interventions when treating a neck or shoulder issue as well as alternative methods, such as craniosacral therapy or yoga. In a pediatric setting, holistic therapists perform traditional feeding roles for children and also offer holistic nutrition and essential oils to encourage children to eat in a safe and age-appropriate manner (Upledger Institute International, 2022).

Suitability for Practice

Occupational therapists can adopt a holistic focus at any point in their career. Therapists can become holistic after years of applying more traditional treatment skills that may not have been as effective as holistic skills. Holistic practice may be ideal for new graduates motivated to learn techniques involving a nontraditional way of thinking to meet patient goals.

These techniques may not have been discussed in their occupational therapy training and may seem "nonscientific." The best way for new graduates or experienced therapists to gain insight into holistic therapy is by taking continuing education courses on related topics. Often during training, therapists will meet physical or other occupational therapists who also are learning holistic treatment skills. These study group connections can provide opportunities to hone the new skills to apply later in a work setting. Most of the growth in attaining holistic knowledge happens outside of work and then is incorporated slowly into patient sessions as therapists master the new skills and their desire to practice them in a work setting increases.

Supervision from holistic occupational therapists can help new graduates interested in the field. More experienced holistic therapists have had extensive practice in not only applying holistic knowledge with varied diagnoses but also with how to document and bill them ethically and appropriately.

References

American Occupational Therapy Association. (2020). Occupational therapy practice framework: Domain and process (4th ed.). *American Journal of Occupational Therapy, 74*(Suppl. 2), 7412410010p1-7412410010p87. https://doi.org/10.5014/ajot.2020.74S2001

Fields, B., & Smallfield, S. (2022). Occupational therapy practice guidelines for adults with chronic conditions. *American Journal Occupational Therapy, 76*(2), 7602397010. doi: https://doi.org/10.5014/ajot.2022/762001

Lubes, M., & Vadnais, E. (2014). *How to become a holistic OT.* Holistic OT. https://holisticot.org/holistic-ot/#:~:text=We%20suggest%20becoming%20educated%20in,healing%2C%20spirituality%2C%20and%20nutrition

Upledger Institute International. (2022). Discover CranioSacral therapy and SomatoEmotional release. https://www.upledger.com/therapies/

Velozo, C. A. (2021). Using measurement to highlight occupational therapy's distinct value. *American Journal of Occupational Therapy, 75*(6), 7406150010. https://doi.org/10.1054/ajot.2021.746001

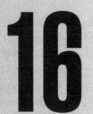

Telehealth

Shelli Dry, OTD, OTR/L, MEd

Telehealth in a Nutshell

Telehealth is an innovative service delivery model used to provide therapeutic services, training, consultation, and assessments when a patient and their health care provider are in different geographical locations. In a 2018 position paper, the American Occupational Therapy Association (AOTA) defined *telehealth* "as the application of evaluative, consultative, preventative, and therapeutic services delivered through information and communication technology" (p. 1). Telehealth also is referred to as *teleintervention* or *teletherapy*.

Telehealth can be delivered synchronously through direct video and audio connectivity or asynchronously through a store-and-forward process. Synchronous services involve a therapeutic intervention in which the provider and patient are connecting via an electronic device at the same time. Both parties communicate directly with each other, and the video allows real-time observations. Common electronic devices for delivering synchronous services include computers, tablets, smartphones, and applications. Options exist for using an online software system that does not require downloading software or an application. With either type of service, end-to-end encryption is a requirement for security. Interactive synchronous services can be delivered individually or in a group setting.

Asynchronous service delivery involves information being transferred between provider and patient at nonspecific times. Patients capture images, events, or data in their location and then store that information briefly before transferring it securely to the provider, who interprets it and decides on the next intervention steps. Using an application to monitor medical devices or a home exercise program are examples of an asynchronous model.

Akselrud, R. (Ed.). *Quintessential Occupational Therapy:*
A Guide to Areas of Practice (pp 171-178).
© 2023 Taylor & Francis Group.

Telehealth benefits include easier access to services, reduced waiting times, improved cost effectiveness and outcome measures, and higher patient motivation (Kairy et al. 2009). Patients who live in a remote environment can reduce costly travel to and from appointments and accessing therapists from home saves time. Allowing providers who live in one state to see a patient in a different state improves patient access to specialists with advanced knowledge related to their condition. Specialists can be consulted easily during a synchronous teletherapy session, and arranging and engaging in cotreatment with both providers logging in simultaneously can improve the continuity of care. Working directly within patient homes allows occupational therapists the opportunity to practice functional activities within this environment at the time they occur, promoting improved generalization of skills.

A meta-analysis comparing the effects of telehealth with traditional face-to-face service delivery has found little difference in outcomes when a single approach was used and a significant improvement in outcomes when cognitive and physical approaches were paired in sessions (Speyer et al., 2018). In addition, outcomes were reached more quickly when occupational therapists therapeutically adapted items in the home to enhance carry over of treatment activities.

Telehealth challenges can include technology interruptions and difficulties with converting hands-on techniques to an online environment, with offering multisensory experiences, and with providing adaptive equipment. Technology interruptions can be adjusted for following some general guidelines in Table 16-1. Occupational therapists can talk patients through their own technology challenges to improve success.

Occupational therapists should be ready to demonstrate techniques on a model or through drawings or handouts. Multisensory environments can be created using items within a patient's home and adapting their use to enhance the sensory experience. It is also possible to arrange a telehealth session to collaborate with an equipment vendor to order the appropriate equipment.

Occupational Therapy's Role

Occupational therapists who choose to use a telehealth model should follow all laws, regulations, and codes of ethics to provide the best possible services for patients. The Center for Connected Health Policy (CCHP) is the national telehealth policy resource center (CCHP, 2020b). CCHP has a compilation of federal and state laws and policies to allow a practitioner access to the most updated regulations (CCHP, 2022a). Practitioners can register with the CCHP to receive updates to laws and regulations. The Uniform Law Commission's Uniform Telehealth Act (2022) establishes a registration process that will allow out-of-state practitioners to deliver services in states that adopt the act as long as they follow standards of care and work within their scope of practice. If working in a state that is different from the therapist's place of residence, it is crucial to identify if that state's laws require a physician's referral. AOTA's state affairs group maintains a resource that outlines regulations, statutes, and regulatory statements by state (AOTA, 2020b).

Telehealth is easily adapted for intervention with patients of all ages. For example, early intervention models using parent-mediated interventions that families can implement with a child have improved treatment efficacy (Criss, 2013). Multiple states use telehealth services for early intervention to decrease the challenges of provider shortages, long travel times, and missed visits for children with weakened immune systems.

In school-age groups, telehealth may utilize direct therapy techniques and include a consultative approach for teacher and paraprofessional training. For example, occupational therapists have the opportunity to attend Individualized Education Program team meetings using video conferencing, thus decreasing travel and time out of the office. Most school-based interventions are easily converted to an online approach, and therapists can offer effective therapy to students using a variety of techniques. Individualized Education Program documentation must indicate that services are being provided via a telehealth platform.

TABLE 16-1

Best Practices for Telehealth

BEFORE SELECTING A TELEHEALTH INTERVENTION

- Consider the complexity of the patient's condition, their ability to be flexible, and their comfort level with the technology.
- Consider the therapist's knowledge, observation skills, and confidence; their ability to be flexible; their comfort level with the technology; and their ability to focus on accountability for functional life skills.

GENERAL CONSIDERATIONS

- Select a low-traffic area in which to set up the technology and hold sessions to ensure patient privacy.
- Mute cell phones and alerts.
- Ensure that the camera, laptop, speakers, and headphones have been fully charged and that a charger and plug are nearby.
- Keep the monitor at eye height with lighting behind the camera and look directly into the camera.
- Wear a headset to keep the conversation private and to improve patient comprehension.
- Have room to move around and switch positions.
- Have a plan for therapist and patient technology issues.
- Keep a foot rest and water nearby. Take stretch breaks and hydrate.

SESSION CONSIDERATIONS

- Be sure the patient and family understands how to adjust their speaker volume.
- Have a clear vision for each session.
- Approach the session as a part of the team dedicated to helping.
- Spend time to build rapport and create a relationship, offering collaboration, support, and agreement.
- Use open-ended questions.
- When converting hands-on techniques, use a model to demonstrate hand placement and techniques for applying pressure, and then help the learning coach or assistant practice the hand placement while demonstrating or describing how to adjust the techniques according to a patient's response.

Telehealth also can be implemented successfully with adults with physical, self-care, social-emotional, and mental health impairments (Forducey, 2012). It can be used in home health, hospitals, veterans' groups, prisons, and mental health settings. Telehealth has been used to successfully rehabilitate individuals recovering from orthopedic conditions, neurological challenges, developmental delays, mental health disorders, and physical limitations.

Evaluation and Assessments

Research has found that telehealth is effective for patients with a variety of conditions; however, this approach is not suitable for everyone (Peretti et al., 2017). Occupational therapists must explore a patient's response to the treatment presentation and use their clinical judgment to decide whether to continue using this model, to switch to a traditional model, or to use a blended approach.

When setting up a treatment session, occupational therapists should consider the role they will play in the session. Therapists may use consultative coaching strategies or direct strategies, depending on a patient's needs and abilities. Many therapists have found that occupation-based frameworks that focus on the person, occupation, and context are adapted easily to telehealth (e.g., Person–Environment–Occupation–Performance Model; Gately et al., 2020; Nissen, 2017). The Person–Environment–Occupation–Performance Model, which has been shown to be a good fit, is a top-down, patient-centered model that considers both intrinsic and extrinsic characteristics and includes individualized therapy sessions, allowing therapists to consider all aspects of a patient's environment and to make changes as needed.

Other occupation-focused frameworks that fit well in this setting include the Model of Human Occupation and the Canadian Model of Occupational Performance and Engagement (Hanson & Magee, 2018; Wong & Fisher, 2015; Zahoransky & Lape, 2020). Occupation-based models should be used to guide therapists' decisions when considering the environment's impact on occupational performance and when considering using occupational adaption to improve all aspects of a patient's health and well-being.

Interventions

Organizing telehealth sessions around a specific model and using a structured format is a recommended best practice. Additional best practices include preparing for the session, verifying the person logged in is the person assigned for therapy, keeping enough flexibility in the schedule to allow patient-centered care, and keeping a structured routine. Preparation for a telehealth session includes reviewing patient charts and other information, identifying a private and quiet location for the session to occur, turning on lights, and charging or plugging in the equipment to be used. Therapists should mute their cell phone, hydrate before the session, and avoid eating or chewing gum. To make eye contact, therapists should look at the camera, not the screen.

For the first telehealth appointment, occupational therapists must confirm that they are speaking to the right person and have patients confirm their date of birth or address. Therapists should explain privacy and confidentiality and what to do if the session is interrupted or the patient needs to take a break. The first session includes developing rapport, teaching the session routines, and engaging in pleasurable activities that focus on patient goals. Therapists provide patients with their contact information and determine patients' preferred methods for receiving reminders and other forms of communication.

For ongoing sessions, occupational therapists begin each session with a greeting and review the prior week's work. Therapists then assess patient needs for the current session and begin preparatory activities to get the mind and body ready for therapy. The middle of the session focuses on goal-related activities, and the end celebrates all achievements, reviews activities and accomplishments from the current day, and plans for the next session.

Electronically mailing or digitally transferring a welcome packet with an intake form that includes scheduling preferences, an informed consent document, and all required authorizations can help therapists organize the materials. Therapists should identify the time and day the information should be returned and provide the family with instructions for logging into the session and running a technology check. Therapists can send an inventory checklist to determine what items are readily available before a session but should be prepared to adjust session plans according to patient needs.

Discharge Planning

Discharge planning includes the decisions that need to be made in order to set up the client for transitioning from one stage to another and could include referrals to other services. An example of transition planning can be a student who no longer meets eligibility for occupational therapy or is in the process of transitioning from junior high to high school (AOTA, 2020c). Discharge planning typically involves reassessment of skills, collaboration with other team members, and communicating the discharge plan with the client and/or the client's family or caregivers.

Additionally, the discharge plan should include client and caregiver education regarding adaptation techniques, utilization of equipment, and environmental modifications. The primary goal of discharge planning is to promote continued health and wellness.

Essential Needs

Practitioners who wish to explore telehealth as a service delivery model will need to ensure they have access to a private location, a high-speed internet service and a quality camera and microphone for their laptop. Practitioners will require access to a Health Insurance Portability and Accountability Act of 1996 and Health Information Technology for Economic Clinical Health compliant platform for their online services and documentation storage. Practitioners who are new to telehealth will also want to identify a mentor who can help them work through challenges and they may want to explore training. The National Consortium of Telehealth Resource Centers (2022) has monthly webinars to support new practitioners and experienced practitioners with the ultimate goal of increasing telehealth adoption. They offer free training and recordings of past education events and outline upcoming events on their webpage.

Informed Consent

Obtaining patients' informed consent is a requirement for telehealth in most geographical areas. This consent is mandated to include the benefits and constrictions or risks of using this service model, a description of the model, and the equipment required. Informed consent should include the security services, including a description of the Health Insurance Portability and Accountability Act of 1996 and the Health Information Technology for Economic and Clinical Health Act security maintenance when the service location is in the United States. When and how consent was obtained should be recorded in the patient's medical records.

Therapy Principles

Understanding and adhering to therapy principles and the practice acts of both the state of the originating site and of the distant site is essential. In cases in which the principles in one state are less restrictive than are those in the other state, occupational therapists must follow the more restrictive requirements. Examples of restrictions include occupational therapists' use of visual-perceptual strategies in treatment or therapists' requirements for additional education before suggesting the use of therapeutic modalities. Therapy principles include following the *Occupational Therapy Code of Ethics* (AOTA, 2020a) and standards for documentation. Regardless of whether the occupational therapy services are being reimbursed or not, the therapist is required to complete all documentation in regard to billing and the provided services through telehealth (AOTA, 2018).

Licensure Laws

Occupational therapists are required to follow all licensure laws from the originating site where the patient is located and the distant site where the therapist is located. AOTA's state licensure document (AOTA, 2020b) can be used for a guide on licensure laws in the United States, as can the World Federation of Occupational Therapists' (2017) document for licensing internationally.

Documentation

Effective documentation for sessions, assessments, consultations, and other services should include a statement that the services were performed via telehealth, the platform used and security requirements followed, and the consent obtained. The telehealth service delivery model follows the same documentation laws and ethics requirements that are mandated for all occupational therapy practice. The intervention plan should include the service location as being online, and the goals should be written to address functional improvements. When discharging a patient from telehealth, the discharge plan should address the reason for discharge and any recommendations the therapist has for the patient including home training programs.

Tips and Advice From the Field

The minimum requirements for providing telehealth include an electronic device with a working camera and microphone and access to the internet. The device needs a minimum of 10 mbps of upload and download speed with a latency of under 300 ms to ensure effective transfer of voice and picture. The preferred upload and download speed is 35 mbps. A faster transfer allows for clearer pictures and voice quality, and the lower latency decreases choppy audio. The internet browser selection can affect service quality, and the browser must allow camera and microphone access for the sessions to occur. To prevent limitations with camera and sound, allow all updates to the internal or external microphone and camera.

To improve session quality, therapists should add an external camera to allow for changes in camera angle, to allow for documents to be reviewed, and to allow for more precise details to be emphasized when demonstrating techniques. A headset is helpful to diminish the potential for the session being overheard and to improve the quality of the sound and patient comprehension when language differences exist. Therapists should be familiar with their computer's accessibility features to allow for patients with visual or hearing difficulties to participate. It also is important to ensure that patients can access these features.

Challenges from poor access to a stable internet provider, with low bandwidth, and with weather-related communication delays are more difficult to control. Table 16-2 details some of the more common errors in telehealth and their trouble-shooting strategies.

There are numerous continuing education courses and special certification training available regarding telehealth and occupational therapy, especially for new graduates.

Table 16-2

Common Telehealth Errors and Solutions

SLOW INTERNET SPEED LEADING TO LATENCY IN SOUND AND POOR PICTURE QUALITY	
Turn off unnecessary programs running in the background	• Skype (Microsoft) connects to the internet even when not in use; quit Skype in the control panel • Dropbox (Dropbox, Inc), Google Drive (Google), and other file synchronization or sharing services run all the time in the background and can reduce internet speed • Cloud backup software is not generally an issue, but shutting it off during sessions can be helpful • Close any unnecessary browsers tabs or windows • If audio is disrupted, replace sound with a phone call or the chat feature
WI-FI SIGNAL DISRUPTION	
Minimize router disruptions	• Hard wire the computer to the router • Move the router closer to the computer location • Use Wi-Fi mesh network systems • Use hotspots when the Wi-Fi signal is disrupted or lost
Manage anti-virus software	• Run software updates during the evening or when no sessions are scheduled
Schedule using the cable internet	• Cable internet is shared by individuals on the same network, which can slow speeds; scheduling sessions during low usage can be effective
Manage delays or disruptions during severe weather	• Patient and provider may not be experiencing the same weather event, so rescheduling or having a backup plan is helpful

References

American Occupational Therapy Association. (2018). Telehealth in occupational therapy. *American Journal of Occupational Therapy, 72*(Suppl. 2), 7212410059p1-7212410059p18. https://doi.org/10.5014/ajot.2018.72S219

American Occupational Therapy Association. (2020a). AOTA 2020 occupational therapy code of ethics. *American Journal of Occupational Therapy, 74*(Suppl. 3), 7413410005p1-7413410005p13. https://doi.org/10.5014/ajot.2020.74S3006

American Occupational Therapy Association. (2020b). *Occupational therapy and telehealth: State statutes, regulations, and regulatory board statements.* https://www.aota.org/-/media/Corporate/Files/Advocacy/State/telehealth/Telehealth-State-Statutes-Regulations-Regulatory-Board-Statements.pdf

American Occupational Therapy Association. (2020c). Occupational therapy practice framework: Domain and process (4th ed.). *American Journal of Occupational Therapy, 74*(Suppl. 2), 7412410010p1-7412410010p87. https://doi.org/10.5014/ajot.2020.74S2001

Center for Connected Healthcare Policy. (2022a). *Resources and reports: State telehealth laws and reimbursement policies report, Fall 2022.* https://www.cchpca.org/resources/category/report-publication-policy-brief/

Center for Connected Healthcare Policy. (2022b). *Welcome to the policy finder.* https://www.cchpca.org/all-telehealth-policies/

Criss, M. J. (2013). School-based telerehabilitation in occupational therapy: Using telerehabilitation technologies to promote improvements in student performance. *International Journal of Telerehabilitation, 5*(1), 39–46. https://doi.org/10.5195/ijt.2013.6115

Forducey, P. G., Glueckauf, R. L., Bergquist, T. F., Maheu, M. M., & Yutsis, M. (2012). Telehealth for persons with severe functional disabilities and their caregivers: Facilitating self-care management in the home setting. *Psychological Services, 9*(2), 144-182. https://doi.org/10.1037/a0028112

Gately, M. E., Tickle-Degnen, L., Trudeau, S. A., Ward, N., Ladin, K., & Moo, L. R. (2020). Caregiver satisfaction with a video telehealth home safety evaluation for dementia. *International Journal of Telerehabilitation, 12*(2), 35-42. https://doi.org/10.5195/ijt.2020.6337

Hanson, S., & Magee, J. (2018). Experiences of occupational therapists working in rural areas of Minnesota and North Dakota. *Occupational Therapy Capstones, 393.* https://commons.und.edu/ot-grad/393

Health Information Technology for Economic and Clinical Health Act, Title XIII of Division A and Title IV of Division B of the American Recovery and Reinvestment Act of 2009, Pub. L. 111-5, codified at 42 U.S.C. §§300jj et seq.; §§17901 et seq.

Health Insurance Portability and Accountability Act of 1996, Pub. L. No. 104-191, §264, 110 Stat. 1936.

Kairy, D., Lehoux, P., Vincent, C., & Visintin, M. (2009). A systematic review of clinical outcomes, clinical process, healthcare utilization and costs associated with telerehabilitation. *Disability and Rehabilitation, 31*(6), 427–447. https://doi.org/10.1080/09638280802062553

National Consortium of Telehealth Resource Centers. (2022). *NCTRC webinar series.* https://telehealthresourcecenter.org/nctrc-webinar-series/

Nissen, R. (2017). *Best practice model for delivery of telehealth occupational therapy services for clients with dementia and their caregivers.* Texas Women's University. https://twu-ir.tdl.org/bitstream/handle/11274/9389/2017Nissen.pdf

Peretti, A., Amenta, F., Tayebati, S. K., Nittari, G., & Mahdi, S. S. (2017). Telerehabilitation: Review of the state-of-the-art and areas of application. *JMIR Rehabilitation and Assistive Technologies, 4*(2), e7. https://doi.org/10.2196/rehab.7511

Speyer, R., Denman, D., Wilkes-Gillan, S., Chen, Y., Bogaardt, H., Kim, J., Heckathorn, D., & Cordier, R. (2018). Effects of telehealth by allied health professionals and nurses in rural and remote areas: A systematic review and meta-analysis. *Journal of Rehabilitation Medicine, 50*(3), 225–235. https://doi.org/10.2340/16501977-2297

Uniform Law Commission. (2022). *Uniform Telehealth Act.* National Conference of Commissioners on Uniform State Laws 2022, Philadelphia, PA, United States.

Wong, S. R., & Fisher, G. (2015). Comparing and using occupation-focused models. *Occupational Therapy in Health Care, 29*(3), 297–315. https://doi.org/10.3109/07380577.2015.1010130

World Federation of Occupational Therapists. (2017). *Working as an occupational therapist in another country.* https://www.wfot.org/resources/working-as-an-occupational-therapist-in-another-country

Zahoransky, M. A., & Lape, J. E. (2020). Telehealth and home health occupational therapy: Clients' perceived satisfaction with and perception of occupational performance. *International Journal of Telerehabilitation, 12*(2), 105–124. https://doi.org/10.5195/ijt.2020.6327

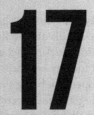

17

Private Practice and Product Development

Robin Akselrud, OTD, OTR/L
and Teresa (Tee) Stock, OTD, MSOT, MBA, OTR/L

Private Practice and Product Development in a Nutshell

A career in occupational therapy can have many paths. As seen in this book, a variety of traditional and emerging areas of practice exist within the field. Lamb (2017) has urged occupational therapy practitioners to "see the growing societal needs and identify paths for the future and actions to move forward" (p. 3). Jacobs (2012) has written about "promOTing occupational therapy through our words, images, and actions" (p. 1). Two paths for creative occupational therapists can be via the exciting opportunities of private practice and product development.

Private practice is when a professional practitioner, such as an occupational therapist, is self-employed and runs their own practice. Occupational therapy private practice began in the 1960s with the expansion of community services and technology. American occupational therapists working in private practice grew from 7.0% to 26.4% in 1990 (McClain et al., 1992).

Occupational therapy private practice in the United States is a $20 billion industry with an annual growth rate of 1.1% and an estimated future growth rate of 1.9% between 2016 and 2022 (Profitable Venture, 2019). As of 2019, at least 60% of all occupational therapists offered private practice services to patients while working other paid jobs (Profitable Venture, 2019). In addition, the 2015 *American Occupational Therapy Association (AOTA) Salary and Workforce Survey* stated that 21% of the respondents would strongly consider and 38% would somewhat consider future private practice.

Akselrud, R. (Ed.). *Quintessential Occupational Therapy:*
A Guide to Areas of Practice (pp 179-183).
© 2023 Taylor & Francis Group.

Many occupational therapists who have a passion for helping others are also creative or business minded. Therapists can effectively use their skills and abilities to help others and earn a primary or secondary income through entrepreneurship and product development. Starting one's own business has pros and cons, and practitioners must fully assess their physical and emotional abilities, risk tolerance, and finances. Although positive aspects of being one's "own boss" include having more flexibility in one's schedule, potentially earning a higher income, and having autonomy, less attractive aspects include having increased stress, challenges managing employees, and difficulty delineating work and personal time.

One approach to view starting a private practice is through a product (service, concept, or physical product) development lens. Product development is defined as being involved in all stages of bringing a product from concept or idea through market release and beyond. The stages may include identifying a need, quantifying the opportunity, conceptualizing the product, validating the solution, building the product roadmap, developing a viable product, releasing the product to users, and responding to feedback (ProductPlan, 2022).

Practitioner Story About Path to Private Practice

(Teresa [Tee] Stock's story): "I had a marketing background and switched careers to become an occupational therapist. I was happily working in school-based practice when another therapy professional asked if I wanted to start seeing some children privately. She explained how she did this and gave advice for how much to charge and how to set it up. Clients were primarily word of mouth and professional peer referrals at first. The local need for in-home therapy in my area was readily apparent, and this part (private practice) of my career expanded. Working privately allowed more flexibility, more autonomy, and a higher pay rate per hour. The families were and still are grateful to have the in-home services and word of mouth continues to grow. As time has gone on, others taught me how to get on insurance plans. I have developed networking groups and found resources through online media and my state and national organizations. I love the flexibility I have and the change I am able to make in my clients' lives through my occupational therapy business."

Potential Areas in Which to Work

Occupational therapists can work in various settings. They can work in schools, community education settings, outpatient clinics, long-term care, hospitals, and early intervention settings. They may also work in home and community settings, mental and behavioral health settings, and academia settings and conduct research (AOTA, 2022). Starting a private practice business on the side or full-time can be done in almost any work setting but should not conflict with other work roles.

Potential Products to Develop

Fred Sammons is perhaps one of the most famous occupational therapy entrepreneurs. He started a small mail order business to earn extra money by selling adaptive devices. Sammons noticed there were needs for certain products and they were not available. He began developing and marketing what was needed for his patients to the greater community (Jacobs, 2012). Sammons went on to be named one of the 100 most influential occupational therapy practitioners of all time (American Occupational Therapy Foundation, 2022).

Karen Jacobs is another renowned occupational therapist who has won numerous occupational therapy awards including the Eleanor Clarke Slagle Lectureship Award. Jacobs is an author, professor, researcher, and entrepreneur. Among her entrepreneurial forays, she has written numerous children's books, developed the journal *WORK*, hosted podcasts, and started an ergonomics business (Boston University College of Health & Rehabilitation Sciences, 2022).

Jan Olsen, founder of Learning Without Tears, launched her business after recognizing the opportunity for an occupational therapy lens on handwriting instruction. She had been volunteering, assisting with handwriting instruction, in her son's classroom and was asked to help more and more students. According to the Learning Without Tears website:

> Responding to John's tears over handwriting in first grade, Jan used her occupational therapy training and background to develop strategies to facilitate his handwriting skills. John's teacher noticed his progress and asked Jan to help other students in the class. Soon, Jan became known in the area as the tutoring solution for handwriting, and her ideas became the basis for the first therapist's guide, *Handwriting Without Tears*. (Learning Without Tears, 2022)

However, many other occupational therapists also think of product ideas that have also launched private practice or been a key part of their occupational therapy life. Some of the products that have been developed include the following:

- Journals (such as *WORK* [Boston University College of Health & Rehabilitation Sciences, 2022; Jacobs, 2012])
- Card decks (activities of daily living/instrumental activities of daily living, yoga, exercise, safety, etc.)
- Books, including children's books (Jacobs, 2012)
- Learning platforms and forums, such as the OT Potential Club and OccupationalTherapy.com
- Assessments
- Curriculum (handwriting, social skills, etc.)
- Therapy materials companies
- Adaptive clothing and devices

Tips and Advice From the Field

Before embarking on an entrepreneurial career or side hustle, first ask the following questions:
- Why do you want to start this new venture?
- Do you have sufficient time to build this venture?
- Are you a self-starter? Do you give up easily? How do you handle failure? Stress?
- What are your business goals for 6 months, 1 year, and 5 years after you begin?

Answer the following questions after determining your personal suitability and goals for this venture:
- What is your niche? Is there a robust market in this area?
- Do you have enough experience in this area? Are there mentors available?
- Are other practitioners working successfully in this area? Are there competitors?
  Key steps to success include the following tasks:
- Compose and follow mission and vision statements for the venture.
- Seek expert advice from an accountant and lawyer to determine the business, legal, and organizational structure.
- Create a business name.

- Conduct a market analysis and choose a geographic location for operations after performing a needs assessment and studying trends.
- Develop business and marketing plans.
- Take relevant continuing education and certification courses.
- Learn and stay current on the ethics and state laws affecting the venture.
- Collaborate with practitioners from occupational therapy and other disciplines.

Finally, following this advice can help you learn from our mistakes (Akselrud & Stock, 2020):

- Start small.
- Document your goals and progress daily.
- Perfect your competitive advantage.
- Utilize students and volunteers.
- Buy and invest in only essential items to start.
- Ask for guidance and help. No one person can do it all!

Most importantly, to be successful, it helps to love what you do.

A competitive advantage is an advantage that a company or therapist has over other competitors in filling a need or function. It is the ability of a company to provide a better value proposition to clients than competitors who provide the same product (Gordon, 2022).

Students and volunteers can help get your private practice going and help you grow it over time. They can be assigned projects, such as research, that may be needed to make your business plan. It is our experience that the students and volunteers may have varied expertise that adds value and provides an opportunity to move forward more quickly with your business plan.

New occupational therapy graduates and even experienced practitioners should gain some experience in the field before starting a new independent venture. Supervision by others and learning through education and clinical and business experiences can help therapists gain more knowledge and expertise and add value to their venture or product.

- Resources:
  - *What if You Don't Want to Deal With Insurance? Tips for Private Practitioners* (AOTA, 2021): https://myaota.aota.org/shop_aota/product/OL8564
  - *Navigating Private Practice: How AOTA Is Supporting You* (Lenhardt & Wright, 2021): https://www.aota.org/publications/ot-practice/ot-practice-issues/2021/navigating-private-practice
- Blogs:
  - *A Day in the Life–Pediatric Private Practice* (Jackson Pena, 2015): http://abbypediatricot.blogspot.com/2015/04/a-day-in-life-pediatric-private-practice.html
  - *Learned Lessons From Starting a Private Practice* (McMurdie, 2016): https://www.clinicient.com/blog/lessons-learned-from-starting-a-private-practice/
- Articles:
  - *Occupational Therapy and Entrepreneurship* (Kuehn, 2020): https://www.aota.org/publications/student-articles/career-advice/entrepreneurship
  - *Resources to Start (and Grow) Your Occupational Therapy Business* (Lyon, 2019): https://otpotential.com/blog/occupational-therapy-business
  - *Entrepreneurial Options: Steps to Consider in Starting a Private Practice* (Harmon, 2014): AOTA account required for access

- ○ *Opening a Private Practice in Occupational Therapy* (Hudgins et al., 2018): https://www.aota.org/~/media/Corporate/Files/Publications/CE-Articles/CE-Article-April-2018.pdf
- ○ *Occupational Therapists in Private Practice* (McClain et al., 1992): https://doi.org/10.5014/ajot.46.7.613
- ○ *Private Practice Sales and Marketing* (Leslie, 2016): AOTA account required for access
- Book:
  - ○ *Business Fundamentals for the Rehabilitation Professional* (Richmond, & Powers, 2009)

References

Akselrud, R., & Stock, T. (2020). *Two practitioners' view on starting a private practice while keeping your day job* [PowerPoint Presentation]. Webinar for AOTA 2020.

American Occupational Therapy Association. (2015). *AOTA Salary and workforce survey*. AOTA Press.

American Occupational Therapy Association. (2021). *AOTA webinar: What if you don't want to deal with insurance? Tips for private practitioners*. https://myaota.aota.org/shop_aota/product/OL8564

American Occupational Therapy Association. (2022). *Practice settings*. https://www.aota.org/practice/practice-settings

American Occupational Therapy Foundation. (2022). *Fred Sammons, PhD (Hon), OT, FAOTA*. https://www.aotf.org/About-AOTF/News/fred-sammons

Boston University College of Health & Rehabilitation Sciences. (2022). *Karen Jacobs, OT, EdD, OTR, CPE, FAOTA*. https://www.bu.edu/sargent/profile/karen-jacobs/

Gordon, J. (2022). *Competitive advantage explained: What is competitive advantage*. The Business Professor. https://the-businessprofessor.com/en_US/business-management-amp-operations-strategy-entrepreneurship-amp-innovation/competitive-advantage)

Harmon, S. (2014). Entrepreneurial options: Steps to consider in starting a private practice. *OT Practice, 19*(9), 8–11.

Hudgins, E., Stover, A., & Walsh-Sterup, M. (2018). Opening a private practice in occupational therapy. *AOTA Continuing Education,*   CE1–CE9.   https://www.aota.org/~/media/Corporate/Files/Publications/CE-Articles/CE-Article-April-2018.pdf

Jackson Pena, H. (2015). *A day in the life: Pediatric private practice*. OT Cafe. http://abbypediatricot.blogspot.com/2015/04/a-day-in-life-pediatric-private-practice.html

Jacobs, K. (2012). PromOTing occupational therapy: Words, images, and actions. *American Journal of Occupational Therapy, 66*(6), 652–671. https://doi.org/10.5014/ajot.2012.666001

Kuehn, J. (2020). *Occupational therapy and entrepreneurship*. American Occupational Therapy Association. https://www.aota.org/publications/student-articles/career-advice/entrepreneurship

Lamb, A. J. (2017). Unlocking the potential of everyday opportunities. *American Journal of Occupational Therapy, 71*(6), 7106140010p1-7106140010p8. https://doi.org/10.5014/ajot.2017.716001

Learning Without Tears. (2022). *Learning without tears history*. https://www.lwtears.com/history

Lenhardt., J., & Wright, M. (2021). *Navigating private practice: How AOTA is supporting you*. American Occupational Therapy Association. https://www.aota.org/publications/ot-practice/ot-practice-issues/2021/navigating-private-practice

Leslie, C. A. (2016). Private practice sales and marketing. *OT Practice, 21*(17), 14–16.

Lyon, S. (2019, April 27). *Resources to start (and grow) your OT business*. OT Potential. https://otpotential.com/blog/occupational-therapy-business

McClain, L., McKinney, J., & Ralston, J. (1992). Occupational therapists in private practice. *American Journal of Occupational Therapy, 46*(7), 613–618. https://doi.org/10.5014/ajot.46.7.613

McMurdie, J. (2016). *Learned lessons from starting a private practice*. Clincient. https://www.clinicient.com/blog/lessons-learned-from-starting-a-private-practice/

ProductPlan. (2022). *What is product development?* https://www.productplan.com/learn/what-is-product-development/

Profitable Venture. (2019). *How to start a private occupational therapy practice business in 14 steps*. https://www.profitableventure.com/starting-a-private-occupational-therapy-business/

Richmond, T., & Powers, D. (2009). *Business fundamentals for the rehabilitation professional* (2nd ed.). SLACK Incorporated.

Financial Disclosures

Dr. Robin Akselrud has no financial or proprietary interest in the materials presented herein.

Dr. Inna Babaeva has no financial or proprietary interest in the materials presented herein.

Dr. James Battaglia has no financial or proprietary interest in the materials presented herein.

Aviva Blaustein has no financial or proprietary interest in the materials presented herein.

Dr. Gioia J. Ciani has no financial or proprietary interest in the materials presented herein.

Dr. Dale A. Coffin has no financial or proprietary interest in the materials presented herein.

Dr. Shelli Dry has no financial or proprietary interest in the materials presented herein.

Dr. Nicole A. Fidanza has no financial or proprietary interest in the materials presented herein.

Melanie C. Frank-Hirsch has no financial or proprietary interest in the materials presented herein.

Dana Fried has no financial or proprietary interest in the materials presented herein.

Dr. Mindy Garfinkel has no financial or proprietary interest in the materials presented herein.

Dr. Melissa K. Gerber has no financial or proprietary interest in the materials presented herein.

Heather Gilbert has no financial or proprietary interest in the materials presented herein.

Clarice Grote has no financial or proprietary interest in the materials presented herein.

Nicola Grun has no financial or proprietary interest in the materials presented herein.

Kristy Gulotta has no financial or proprietary interest in the materials presented herein.

Henry Hanif has no financial or proprietary interest in the materials presented herein.

Brett Herman has no financial or proprietary interest in the materials presented herein.

Dr. Yu-Pin Hsu has no financial or proprietary interest in the materials presented herein.

Dr. Douglene Jackson has no financial or proprietary interest in the materials presented herein.

LoriBeth Kimmel has no financial or proprietary interest in the materials presented herein.

Dr. Ivelisse Lazzarini has no financial or proprietary interest in the materials presented herein.

Dr. Catherine J. Leslie has no financial or proprietary interest in the materials presented herein.

Rachelle Lydell has no financial or proprietary interest in the materials presented herein.

Dr. Jacqueline Ndwaru McGlamery has no financial or proprietary interest in the materials presented herein.

April O'Connell has no financial or proprietary interest in the materials presented herein.

AnneMarie O'Hearn has no financial or proprietary interest in the materials presented herein.

Dr. Heather Page has no financial or proprietary interest in the materials presented herein.

Michelle M. Rampulla has no financial or proprietary interest in the materials presented herein.

Miriam Ringel has no financial or proprietary interest in the materials presented herein.

Taylor Skoller has no financial or proprietary interest in the materials presented herein.

Dr. Esty Spitzer has no financial or proprietary interest in the materials presented herein.

Dr. Teresa (Tee) Stock has no financial or proprietary interest in the materials presented herein.

Kelsey Swope has no financial or proprietary interest in the materials presented herein.

Miriam Wachspress has no financial or proprietary interest in the materials presented herein.

Lee Westover has no financial or proprietary interest in the materials presented herein.

Anna Wold has no financial or proprietary interest in the materials presented herein.

Index

Printed in the United States
by Baker & Taylor Publisher Services